"Send forth thy sickle and reap;
for the hour of reaping is come...."

Revelation 14:15

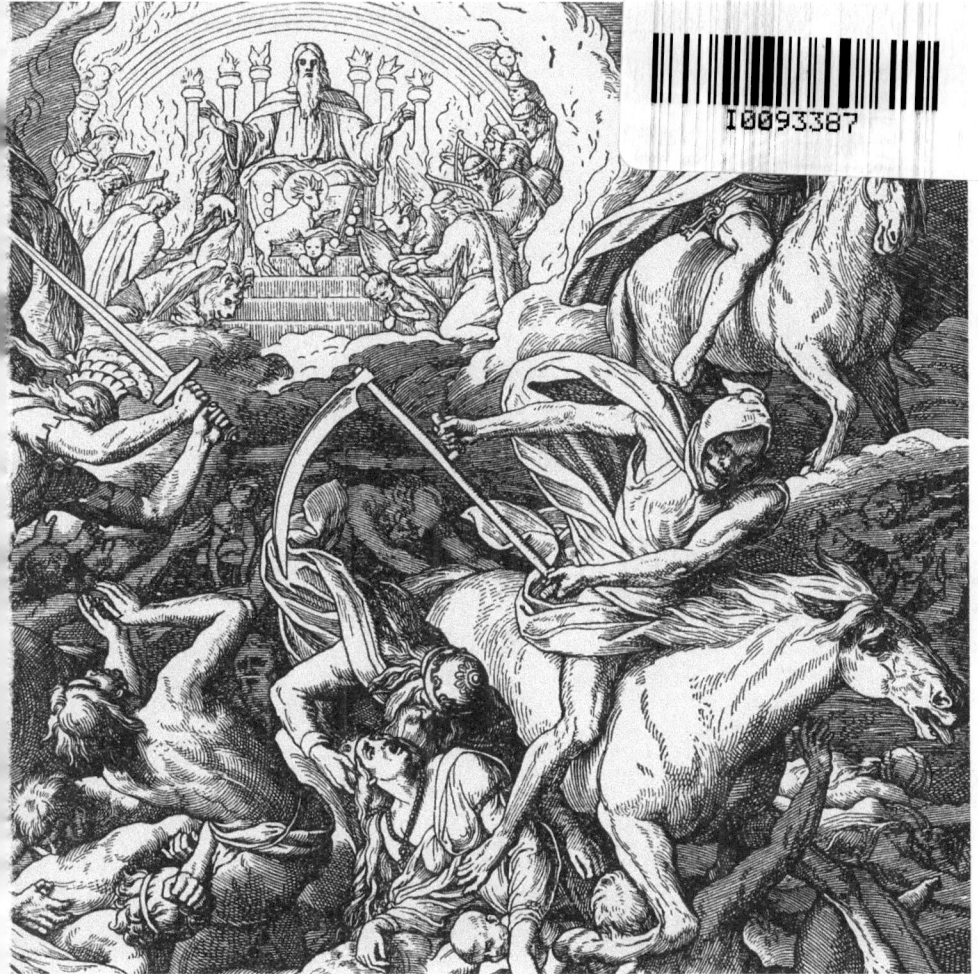

Julius Schnorr von Carolsfeld

The Freak Miracle Trilogy — Book I
Freak Fall: Into the Apocalypse

FREAK FALL

Into the Apocalypse

A novel by Dave Cheadle

Headwaters Christian Resources

Scripture quotations marked (NIV) are taken from the Holy Bible, New International Version®, NIV®. Copyright © 1973, 1978, 1984, 2011 by Biblica, Inc.™ Used by permission of Zondervan. All rights reserved worldwide. www. zondervan.com The "NIV" and "New International Version" are trademarks registered in the United States Patent and Trademark Office by Biblica, Inc.™

Headwaters Christian Resources
PO Box 175, Englewood, CO 80110

www.FreakFall.com
Cover art by Evan D. Cheadle
Book design by Joe Anderson

ISBN: 978-0-9679622-9-0
September 2015

10 9 8 7 6 5 4 3 2 1

To the One who is, who was, and who is to come—
the Wildly-Imaginative Author of His-Story

"Woe to those who call evil good
  and good evil,
who put darkness for light
  and light for darkness,
who put bitter for sweet
  and sweet for bitter.
....

The mountains shake,
  and the dead bodies are like refuse in the streets.
Yet for all this, his anger is not turned away,
  his hand is still upraised."

Isaiah 5:20, 25 (NIV)
....

Then I saw another angel flying in midair, and he had the
eternal gospel to proclaim to those who live on the earth—
to every nation, tribe, language and people.

He said in a loud voice, "Fear God and give him glory,
because the hour of his judgment has come.
Worship him who made the heavens, the earth, the sea
and the springs of water."

Revelation 14:6-7 (NIV)

PROLOGUE:

I made the national news. Fifteen minutes of fame, then back under a rock.

Several times.

Nobody remembers me, because even with five microphones jammed in my face, the cameras were always really on him. On Freak. He was the story. Still is.

Like most high school English teachers, I'm a bit of a hypocrite. I'm quick to lecture students about the joys of writing, but I myself prefer the ease and easy gratification of a quick read. I drove up into the snowy Rockies that March weekend for the good life, expecting to do a little snowshoeing and to savor an unhealthy assortment of craft beers. And to lose myself into an adventure story... not write one.

Looking back, it's a grin to see how one of CNN's top five headlines of the year virtually landed in my lap.

Beyond the laughable ironies, I find the realities of the past few months profoundly unnerving. With the economy in free fall, with institutions collapsing, and with the escalation of fear, disasters and violence... people are frightened. And they are desperate for answers.

For rational explanations. For reliable prophecies.

For hope.

Almost the whole world is waiting to hear more from Freak.

And right now, he's not talking.

Freak says that it's my turn to speak. He says that I must be brutally honest. About him. About myself. About what I've seen. And about how the world—and churches—have been handling all of this global shaking.

If I had my way, I'd turn this assignment over to someone else. Probably Saundra. She would do a good job. She'd knock it out of the park. Saundra's got a degree in journalism. She has covered big-time disasters before. And she actually believes that she has seen some of these angels and demons and all of that.

But, again, Freak insists that the story has fallen to me—it's mine to tell.

So I'd better get on with it.

DARK 1 MAMAS

On Denver's 850 KOA NewsRadio, the Friday morning weather update boasted of 10 inches of fresh powder up around the Divide. Although I'm not a fanatical skier, I do love to clamp on a pair of bear paw snowshoes and go tramping around the Loop Trail a few time each season.

Getting that much snow just in time for spring break... I never gave it a second thought. Between bagels, I told my housemate that he could have the guys over and they could crank up the March Madness games until the shutters flapped. I gave him my bracket, naming which teams would win and lose, told him why, and then gave him a few hundred bucks to place my bets. As usual, I promised him 10 percent of the spoils.

Then I remembered to call Heather. I told her I was headed for the snowy woods and a quiet path less beaten. Told her I needed a little "me" time, alone.

After dismissing my last class on Friday, I busted straight home. I threw together a quick duffle, grabbed my latest book purchase from Amazon, then headed up to our family cabin far off the highway deep within the unsullied solitude of the White River National Forest.

Despite the massive snow dump, I-70 was blow-dry clean from heavy traffic the entire 90 minute drive up from Denver. Eisenhower Tunnel was pretty clogged at Loveland Pass, but otherwise I made surprisingly good time. I felt the yuck of the city melting off my red Expedition as I pumped the big SUV's brakes and rolled down the grade to Dillon Lake and one of the most breathtaking, sun-drenched ski basin valleys in the world.

At the base of the mountain, I peeled off the Interstate.

I timed it well through Silverthorne's three main lights, then started the gradual descent along the Blue River on Highway 9.

At the edge of town, I wheeled into the Last Stop Liquors parking lot. Mountain towns, especially in ski country, are always desperate for parking spaces. Last Stop, nestled in the shadows of four of the busiest ski resorts in Colorado, is forced to more or less share a plowed gravel parking pad with a much older and more neglected establishment: Dillon's Blue River Bible Church.

Blue Bible has been in the valley even longer than the three generations that our family has owned the cabin. In town, complaints against the church are legion, many concerning their oversized historic steeple bell and the congregation's propensity to ring it insanely loudly at ungodly times. It always seems to hammer on bizarre occasions, like Halloween and Fat Tuesday, and at absurd hours, like Sunday mornings before noon.

Two men, one with thick black-rimmed glasses and a shaggy salt-and-pepper beard, stood in dirty Carhartt bib overhauls. They were fussing with a spade and ax between the liquor store and the church. A short third man swayed between them, waving his arms, directing the operation. The subject of their efforts was an enormous new sign, but it was unclear as to whether they were extracting or implanting the exoticism, which declared in huge red block letters:

"PREPARE YOUR ESCAPE."

Then, in smaller letters, "Escape For Tonight — *Park Over There.*" An arrow pointed in my direction, at the liquor store.

Beneath that, "Escape Forever — *Park Right Here,*" with an arrow pointing towards their little rattle-trap white church bus rusting near the chapel's front door.

I sat a moment, mentally unpacking the message, trying to decide if it was clever or insulting.

Still considering the matter, I unbuckled my seatbelt and climbed out. I gave them a last look, then headed towards the familiar glass door graced by a tiny silver bell above the frame.

It's a happy little ringer—it jingles the same greeting for all, sinner and saint alike.

"Anything new?" I asked.

The 20-something blonde sitting at the register wore a crisp whiskey logo cap with a matching vest, unzipped. She was gorgeous, knew it, and apparently didn't mind being reminded of as much by my smile.

She slipped down from her stool and leaned into the counter.

"More trouble," she smiled, "more fighting in the Middle East." She gestured toward the small television screen suspended from the ceiling beside a matching security monitor. "Promises of peace. Rumors of war."

"Spare me," I chuckled. "I'm more into current breweries than current events."

"I thought so," she laughed. "You've been in here before."

She reached past a fat fishbowl of schnapps shooters on the counter to a small beer display. "We've got this seasonal craft brew in from Fort Collins." She patted the colorful carton. "It's on special."

She grinned. "But take a look at these."

I followed her retreating hand past her vest to its new destination, chest high, due west, wagging at the nearest cooler. Sure enough, off the tip of her finger were two racks filled with a set of colorful labels I'd never seen.

"Local," she said. "They just opened a new brewpub on the marina drive down by the reservoir. They're calling the company 'Dillon Beach Brewing.' Ten bucks is a lot for a six-pack, but everyone says they're worth it."

"What's up with the church sign?" I asked, stepping to the cooler.

"City stuff. Code issues. The church never pulled a permit. And they never got a waiver. Their sign is way too big for this end of the valley."

"Hmm." I was taking stock of the labels. They were luscious and inviting. Far more appealing than the obnoxious sign in the stark lot outside.

I opened the cooler and withdrew a long-necked chocolate milk stout. The label said "Cold Dark Mama." The model on the label appeared more Swedish than African. "Dark" apparently referred to the slinky black dress she'd been poured into. And her stilettos. And, I suppose, the beer sloshing around inside the bottle.

I looked closer.

She was stunning. I glanced at the other labels. The same signature woman graced them all, from pale ales to black stouts. Painted in a flashy CGI style that blended cartoon and photograph. Different studio backdrops, but every label with the same profile and wink. Seductive. High glamour. Only slightly comic.

"Nice," I whispered. "I'd love to see more of you in the funny pages."

"My uncle used to say that."

I glanced up, surprised she'd heard.

"Whenever he was leaving, he'd say that: 'See you in the funny pages.'"

I shook my head. "Right. I used to hear it from my grandpa. It took me a while to figure out what a tease he was. I think the joke was a WWII thing."

I turned the bottle and noted a promising 8% alcohol content. I rolled it back to the model. A shapely white thigh spilled through a slit running half way up her hip.

Bare shoulders foamed up from a plunging fur-trimmed collar. She hoisted a tempting bottle in one hand, an overflowing glass in the other.

The clerk shifted, smirking.

I blinked. Sure enough.

"That's you, eh?"

"Wondered if you'd notice." She beamed. "My boyfriend does freelance silk screening and acrylics up the valley in Frisco. He designed it. It's not me... and it is. My boss is an idiot. He still hasn't figured it out."

She paused, calculating.

"Every boss is an idiot," I encouraged. A boyfriend? Hmm.

"My boss doesn't even know. Sales go bonkers whenever I'm on the clock. He's talking about giving me a raise." She winked. "Some customers see it. Some feel it. Magic works either way. What do you think?"

"I think you've got a damn lucky boyfriend."

She wriggled, then looked to the door. Then back at me.

"My boyfriend... he says these labels—and some of the other stuff we've done—are his ticket to the big time. He's building an amazing portfolio. Some of the other art isn't as conservative as what you see here in the store."

My heart skipped.

"We're going to publish the collection when we're done. That'll get him a job in Denver. I'm his ticket out of here. And he's mine."

"You don't like the mountains?"

"I grew up here. Summit County is nice. But there aren't a lot of options out here in the woods. I wanna try the city. What about you... you're from Denver, right?"

"I'm just heading up the hill a few miles." I tipped my head north. "My family has a place off Bootlegger Lake. I'm four-wheeling up to the cabin as soon as I've got my beer. Tomorrow morning, I'll be out there snowshoeing on the Loop."

"Sounds peaceful. A cabin, eh?"

I glanced up at the security monitor.

"Hey," I laughed. "You're on television. Is this a reality show, or what?"

"You guessed it. Please remember to sign the release form before you leave. Without a signature, we'll be forced to cut you from this scene."

The video screen auto-cycled to an elderly couple in the back corner quietly selecting wines.

"Your boyfriend," I said. "the Frisco Kid. I hope he knows how to treat a movie star."

She gave her hair a breezy toss and laughed. "For what it's worth, he's the jealous type. You remind me a bit of him. He's a little older, like you. He's tall, but he's a mountain man... he almost never shaves. And he's a sports stud. He's practically a professional snowboarder."

"You know," I said, tugging on my bare chin, "I used to be a jock. There's nothing like a good game of ball. But I thought you said your boyfriend was an artist?"

"That, too." She stuffed an empty hand into a tight jean pocket and leaned back, rolling her shoulders as if stretching out a kink.

"He is. He's everything. My boyfriend is an artist. A sponsored boarder. A construction worker in the summer. My ticket out of here...." Her gaze dropped, unexpectedly. She began straightening the counter. I decided maybe she was a little shy after all.

A couple of college kids stepped forward to make a purchase, so I drifted back to the cooler. I settled on a six of Dark Mamas, and a second six of Dillon's Wicked Wheat. As I returned to the register, she checked to see which ones I'd pulled.

"These look good," I said, sliding the dream packs across the counter to the real deal.

"That's what they say."

"Listen," I said. "If the reality show doesn't work out, something else will. I'll bet you've got more options than you think. For a girl like you, there's probably at least one golden ticket that comes through this door every week."

She met my gaze.

"I don't want just a season pass or any old scratch ticket... I want to win the Power Ball."

She swallowed awkwardly. "Those Dark Mama's have been selling the best. Guys can't seem to get enough."

"If they're that good, maybe I'll come back in a couple days to grab some more."

She pulled a bag out from beneath the counter and popped it open with a practiced snap. She hesitated, her hand resting on the neck of the nearest Dark Mama.

"Maybe you should grab two more now," she winked. "It'd be a shame if we sold out and you drove back here for nothing."

"For nothing?" I laughed.

I turned and selected another pair of sixes from the cooler. She set the bag aside and retrieved an empty beer flat for what she had deftly upgraded to a full-case purchase.

As I slid the two additions across the counter, I couldn't help my grin.

"You enjoy this, huh? Guys getting all weak-kneed and loading up on these? Doesn't it get a little weird sometimes?"

She nestled the four sixes into the low-cut box, never looking up.

"It's a job. It's okay."

"I think it's more than a job." I laughed. "You've put some skin into the game."

"Like I said, we've got a plan." She met my eyes, not at all defensive. "We're tracking the sales. That'll be part of our pitch with the artwork... something we can leverage to help seal a deal."

"Well, good for you," I said. "I hope you make it big."

"Whatever it takes." She paused for me to pull out my wallet. "You're right, though. It can get a little weird with some of the guys who like to gawk."

"Was I weird?"

"Naw. You were cool. It's all kinda supposed to be a joke anyway. It's the ones who think it's serious that spook me. It gets to feeling like I'm trapped in their eyes."

I opened my billfold and checked for cash.

"What's hard," she added, tossing her head towards the church, "is working every day next to that looney farm. It's gotten even worse since they hired their new pastor from Florida. He storms in here every few days to throw a fit about our advertising. Especially the new sign that we're field testing over there." I followed her nods to a gap between the wall coolers. "I guess the picture must drive him a little schizo."

I followed her nods to a gap between the wall coolers. My eyes took an inventory of where she was pictured on the wall, poster sized, strategically draped in a brewpub advertising towel. Her voluptuous cartoon double wore nothing more than a thin bikini and a wry grin. Her right hand pressed a Wicked Wheat against the mast of a small sailboat. Her other hand held the branded beach towel, clutched by a single corner. She winked as a snow-capped mountain range poked at the distant sky far behind.

"Those folks," she sighed, "can really get creepy whenever they see a little skin."

I pulled my credit card, for the first time not sure what to say.

As I left, the little silver bell tinkled overhead, and I thought I heard her softly call, "See you in the funny pages."

She had no idea.

Then again, neither did I.

THE 2 FALL

Sweet, leisurely Saturday morning coffee. Then a box of juice and a bottle of water into each pocket. A couple of granola bars for the trail, and I was off.

Snowshoeing above 9,000 feet in ten inches of powder is always a lot of work under a spring sun, and it had been a while since I'd been out. Normally, a person would select a long and fairly narrow shoe for navigating deep fluff. The technique would be a bit like cross-country skiing, a shuffle and float across the snow. But, because I like to wander off the beaten trail, I often opt for bear paws. Paws are perfect for underbrush and steeper grades. The disadvantage is how bear paws tend to sink and sometimes toe grab on the upstroke.

I managed to steam up my polarized Oakleys in less than ten minutes. I took them off a few times to smudge off the fog and drips. And I stopped a few times for water and nibbles, or to suck in a good vista treat.

By mid-morning I was back at the cabin, relaxing on the back deck.

Hungry, tired, content.

I took another long hit, my thumb in my book, my mind drifting back to the liquor store checkout and the girl on the towel for the Dillon Beach brew.

Last night, I'd stopped drinking straight from the bottle after my first swig. As advertised, the beer was tasty, worthy of a fine glass.

Now again this morning, I was pouring into my favorite tall mug. I'd started with a pair Wicked Wheats, then quickly matched the score in Dark Mamas in less than an hour.

They foamed and went down marvelously, as expected.

Above, the Colorado sky was an amazing shade of ice blue you never see at lower altitudes or in the city. A few plumes of jet exhaust streaked the sky, billowing from fresh tight ends to wispy fading oblivion far behind. The air was still and the forest quiet, save the occasional plop and rustling sounds from mounds of snow slipping free off low-sagging boughs, then springing high in quick release.

I cracked my paperback's spine and pressed it open, guts down, onto the glass deck table. I reached beneath the table beside my booted foot, groped along the frigid deck, then delivered up from the shadows another frosty Black Mama. She winked at me, now basking in the glorious sun.

Had I known what was up, and what was about to come down, I would have gone in and made a sandwich. Instead, I relished the morning's escape, settling into the irresponsibility and freedom of it all. Not a student, a parent, nor an administrator within a hundred miles. The vast clear sky overhead, the forest, my happily weary legs, the intoxicatingly thin air. And a rich brew getting right to it on an empty stomach.

Life was good.

I studied the label again, more closely than ever.

She was indeed amazing.

I wiped a bead of condensation from the label, rifling a file of mental images as I flicked the moisture from my fingertip into the thin mountain air.

Which was better: her in the flesh, or her on the label?

I lifted the bottle opener, snapped the cap, then rashly emptied another dark brew. Half the milk stout roiled up from the mug's bottom, then rolled down over the lip.

Life, indeed. The good life.

I slid the empty bottle to join the others at the center of the table. Two Wheats, now three Darks, all lined neatly, facing me in a row, each with a grin that sucked me in.

To my left, another plop and rustling swoosh. Another pine shucking a few pounds of a heavy load.

Playing chess with my little chorus line, I moved a Dark from one end of the row to the other, then shuffled a few more, choreographing a perfect balance that now alternated evenly between Darks and Wheats.

A distant jet caught my ear. I glanced to the sky.

Near the ragged snowcapped horizon of the Gore Range, the plane was tiny, but distinct in the clear abyss, descending towards Denver. I could almost see windows. I wondered if anyone might be looking down, seeing the cabin roof, or even my tire tracks in the driveway's snow. Maybe a quick speck, a white flicker of reflected sun bouncing from my table? They wouldn't see me, of course. I was too small. Too nothing. Did not exist.

I adjusted my sunglasses and titled my head for a better view.

I squinted into the sky, watching them inch in my direction, knowing right where they were... and right where they were headed. Knowing that in less than an hour they would be walking down the concourse at Denver International Airport.

Within a margin of error of less than five feet, I could picture the floor pattern where they would be stepping off from the escalator that siphoned passengers up from underground train into the expansive ground floor main terminal. I could see the exact bathroom—the tiled wall art and the white sinks and the metal hand blowers many of the men would use before snagging their luggage from a conveyor at a baggage claim island.

And they knew nothing of me.

My gaze settled back to the bottles. She was frozen, transfixed. I could stare, study every curve, but she couldn't so much as finish her wink. Didn't even know she was being watched.

Hmm. I rolled my head and cracked my neck.

I took off my shades and glanced away to let her breathe.

I imagined someone from the plane with binoculars watching me move the bottles around like chess pieces, like toys. I suddenly felt a little dizzy, and the whole project somehow lost its appeal.

I steadied my hand and pulled an empty from the middle of the row. I rolled it a few times, then slid my fingers up the side and clutched it by the neck.

With a quick hard flick, the bottle went spinning. End-over-end, like a carnival knife. My release felt clean and perfect, and the bottle buried itself with a hollow thunk in a snowdrift some six steps away. Its dark round bottom was a full blood moon, staring back from the exact spot I'd intended.

I snagged another empty.

In a single fluid motion, I flipped the second bottle, this time harder than the first, forcing it from my hand to the unblinking brown eye.

Missed by several inches.

Reached for another of the empties. Tried again.

Sometimes you can release from the foul line and not have to look. It's just the ball and the net from the very instant you let go. You know it. You can feel it in the follow through. You don't even have to watch.

The dark moon base exploded. A hundred tiny razor shards shattered loose, radiating from a direct hit.

Glass and label annihilated.

I shook my head. Surprised, but not. I reached for another bottle. No regrets for labels lost.

I tested its balance and weight, swirling the last half swallow I'd left behind. My gaze again drifted to the sky.

The jet was now directly overhead, trailed by a silver plume feathering behind like a fading ghost.

"You, up there," I whispered. "Watch this."

But before I could turn from the sky, there was a brilliant little flash. Then, a moment later, a much bigger explosion.

And the plane just disappeared.

It took a second to register.

A moment for me to believe.

Gone.

Yet there was the proof. The unmistakable line of a jet exhaust cloud, a white contrail. A declaration of truth in that brilliant sky. And then, at the sharp end of the statement overhead, an abrupt, heart-stopping exclamation point.

I fumbled for my sunglasses. Then looked again.

Now, remember, I'd had a few drinks.

The sun was biting bright, and I might have had a few spots of steam or scratches on my Oakleys, so I'm not saying that what I saw is exactly what was. Nor am I saying what I did afterwards is exactly right. They tell me the first few times I told this part, it was a little different every time. I'm almost to the point now where I worry that I remember how to tell the story better than I can recall the actual events.

When I looked back up, I remember my eyes shooting right back to the head of the silver jet cloud. It took some squinting, but I think I saw a bit of a drifting starburst or smoke or lit-up oxygen or something, with some darker streams trailing down and tapering out almost immediately. It was a bit like the wispy cloud puff that you see from a bottle rocket that explodes at the highest edge of view.

Straining for all I was worth, I seemed to be able to make out a few chunks of plane or something falling at incredible speeds.

Within moments, stuff just started spontaneously popping into existence from out of nowhere. All different sizes, dropping so fast I couldn't really make out the shapes and decipher what anything was. It was totally surreal. Later, they said some of it was luggage, some of it was pieces of plane, and of course, some of it was body parts and people strapped to chairs.

I stood, mesmerized and horrified, the air deathly still, junk blooming out of the cold blue and screaming down into the valley around me. I don't remember the sound of the jet's explosion ever making its way to me. It might have. Maybe I was in shock. Maybe it was the beer.

Suddenly, there was this one black dot heading straight towards me. It grew so fast I almost wanted to raise my arms against it. Then, the second before it disappeared with a crash into some very nearby trees, it looked to be a body.

Intact. Spread eagle.

It busted into the pines not fifty yards up the steep mountain pitch above my deck.

Stunned, I locked onto a landmark tree where I thought it must have hit. Then I looked up to see if anything else might be headed my way. Debris, all sizes, was still hailing down all around the valley, but nothing else fell anywhere near my cabin.

Then it was over.

Whoever it was, they had to be dead. Probably pooling in a bloody splat. The investigators would have one heck of a time digging through snow and bagging the remains.

I relocated the landmark pine, judged how deep the snow was, then wished the corpse had fallen either closer or farther away. I stepped off the deck and started making my way up the hill. By the time I was in the shade of the thick woods, I was plunging and wading through several feet of snow. I had to turn back.

Normally, I can slip in and out of my snowshoes like lightning. Now, I fumbled with buckles and straps and could hardly tell what I was doing. By the time I grabbed my hat and gloves and launched into the undergrowth and pines the second time, I was sweating heavily and having difficulty remembering exactly which route I should be holding to make it to that tallest ponderosa. The forest grew thicker and the increasingly steep grade of my climb quickly began taking its toll. My head was reeling, and I wished I'd gone to the kitchen in between the bottles I'd so hurriedly emptied. I should have made a lunch and swallowed some water to mix with all of the beer I'd dumped into a dry stomach.

Of course, if I'd been inside the cabin, then I wouldn't have seen the explosion. I doubt I would have heard the body crashing through the branches. It might have been spring before anyone even knew where he had burrowed his grave.

All the recent snow made the forest a marshmallow fairyland of puffy white mounds. Mounds on the sagging boughs, mounds on small bent trees in patches of undergrowth, and mounds stacked high on a few protruding stumps and fallen logs. It was easier than I expected to spot the anarchy and riot of disturbed snow and cracked ponderosa limbs that marked where flesh had fled the heavens and returned to earth.

Again, I wondered if I had any business approaching the scene.

I shuffled closer, fighting my way up the increasingly difficult ascent.

A deep messy hole punched the snow near the rough trunk of that battered, freakishly large specimen of a pine. The body had plowed through a net of branches, bringing a few down with it. Thankfully, no blood... I hate blood. Piles of snow dumped from the shaken tree littered the entire scene. A torn scrap of jacket dangled from one of the conifer's lower branches above the death pit, morbidly draped among the broken limbs. I shuddered, debating my retreat.

The incline rose even steeper between me the hole. Wearing snowshoes, there was no way I could climb the sharp pitch to get any closer to the massive trunk. If I took them off, I'd probably sink at least three or four feet into a winter's worth of snow. A mountain rescue team would carry a sled and all the equipment needed to retrieve the corpse with ease. I'd let them handle this.

I glanced around for some way to flag the area. If it started snowing again, the investigators might need a marker to find the right spot.

Near my feet, I spied a white aspen branch. It was a hefty thickness, rising from a drift, pointing almost straight up. It would do. I decided to pull it out from the snow and lodge it sideways into the branches of the big pine. I gave the limb a tug.

It wouldn't budge. It must have been attached to a fallen tree deep below. I surveyed the snow, trying to judge which direction the Aspen trunk was lying so I could manage the right leverage to break the branch free.

Scanning the white terrain, something was wrong.

Globs of snow had shaken loose from many of the surrounding trees. Craters from the dropped piles were scattered everywhere. Here at my feet, though, the disrupted surface was not sunken or pocked. The surface was elevated, swollen upwards from below. A straight long mound was pushed up like a mole-run in a field. The unlikely formation flowed directly from my feet to the big hole at the base of the pine.

The victim had dropped there, then slid here.

I was practically standing on what I supposed was a mangled, stiffening cold cadaver.

Again, keep in mind I'd been drinking. Heavily. On an empty stomach. My head was buzzing, and I really don't know what came over me. I do remember trying to dig with my hands, then taking off my snowshoes. My feet and legs sank deeper than expected. I grabbed one of my snowshoes and began digging, tossing snow with it like I had a shovel. I kept scooping the bowl bigger because snow caved in from the sides.

I've got no idea how long it took. Investigators said I dug down almost six feet, past the fresh powder and all the way into the hard pack from last October.

I kept digging and digging. Exhausted, I still couldn't stop. I had to get the hole big enough for me to be able to work the snowshoe, and wide enough for me to be able lift the body out. Finally, I hit something semi-hard, and I knew it was the victim.

How, I don't know, but I starting pitching snow like a madman. I scraped the bottom of the pit in a flurry of strength that came from who knows where. The sides continued caving, and I was afraid I was standing on the guy. Or that he'd get buried again if I paused to rest.

I was onto a human for sure, a body in a thick parka. But I couldn't tell which way he was lying, or even if he was facing right-side up or upside-down. All I kept getting was jacket. I could hardly see through my sweat and foggy sunglasses. Like an idiot, it took me forever to think to throw the glasses off.

When I looked down again, my vision finally cleared.

"Oh, God."

I recoiled like a drunken snake.

Eventually, I steadied myself for a longer look.

A face.

The entire left side, ripped open.

His eyes were closed, and I could see frayed cheek muscle and white bone through several sickeningly deep gashes. Blood was pooling and seeping around his head, yet somehow he looked at rest like nothing I'd ever seen. That was the most eerie thing about the whole ordeal. He appeared happy. Content. With a look like that, I knew he had to be dead.

To this day, nobody has officially said whether it was my snowshoe that laid open his face, or if it was the branches that had done the damage. Maybe we'd each done our part. Either way, my mind holds a terrible snapshot of his face that I wish I could forget. I've mostly played along with the published reports that blamed it on the trees. People have been very kind about this, but I'll probably wonder for the rest of my life. Why didn't I pull off those stupid glasses sooner? Why didn't I slow down and be more careful when I knew I'd come to the body?

It could be that in my addled brain, I figured he was dead already, and it wouldn't matter.

But if I thought he was dead, why did I dig so furiously?

As clearly as I can recall the haunting image, I'm equally unclear about how I dragged him up from the hole. Nor can I remember when or how I decided for sure he was alive.

At some point I had my snowshoes back on, and I was tugging and pulling him down to my cabin. Then I had him face up on my deck to confirm faint wisps of steam from his shallow breathing. I knew he would be dead for sure by the time anyone could drive up and haul him out, so somehow I wrangled him into the back end of my SUV and raced down the hill to the Trauma Center in Frisco.

I ran through lights and laid on my horn all the way into the parking lot. A bunch of people mobbed me from the brick two-story building the moment I skidded to a stop.

Thankfully, mountain hospitals are equipped for ski wrecks and avalanche rescues. This wasn't the first time they'd had to deal with someone who'd hit hard or been buried alive. They dealt with broken bones, frostbite and hypothermia every day.

A lot of what happened gets hazy here, and some of this comes from what I've read and what others have told me. I guess I'd driven down without any ID. I puked and passed out for a minute or two before they got me to the door. The other guy was in a parka and obviously wasn't talking, so they jumped to the conclusion that we'd been backcountry skiing. They assumed we had gotten drunk over lunch, and then we'd screwed up on our way back to the SUV and run into a tree. That stuff happens all the time. For them, this was just another Summit County day in the ER.

Things didn't get crazy until someone checked the patient's wallet and pieced together that in spite of the fact he was wearing a winter parka, he might have dropped from the plane.

Then some college student with a sprained ankle in the ER reached down and pulled a cell phone from his boot.

He shot 90 seconds of video, managing to catch one of the hospital volunteers recognizing the victim and shouting a name.

The kid posted his clip before anyone realized what he'd done, and the word was out.

+ DAVE CHEADLE +

THE H3SPITAL

I woke up taped to an IV in a white bed. They were leaving me alone at the edge of the ER, but there was a flurry of chaos out in the lobby. A mob of staff was scrambling around behind a curtain at the back end of the big room.

Then someone noticed my lifted head and my fluttering eyes. Suddenly, they swarmed at me like bees.

Security and a man in scrubs drove them off. Someone latched onto my bed and wheeled me down the hall into a darkening black tunnel.

When I came to again, I was in a private room. A Summit County Deputy Sheriff stood by the window, looking back and forth between me and the raucous crowd growing outside in the parking lot.

For ten minutes or so, I pretended to be sleeping, sneaking squints as much as I dared. Trying to inventory the room, to review what had happened. To determine what the heck was going on.

From my angle, the sheriff's gun and holster were at eye level, and they seemed a lot bigger and more out of place in that hospital room than I would have thought. The sheriff's eyes were dark, set deep between a thick mustache and bushy black brows on a serious face. His hairy forearms were muscular, with sharp definition below a navy short sleeve shirt loaded with patches, badges and a treasure chest of service bling. His duty jacket was draped over the room's only chair. The navy stripe on the side of his gray trousers kept drawing my eye back to his holster.

I gathered my wits as best I could, trying to connect the dots between the plane explosion, the guy I dug from the snow, and the weapon a few steps from my forehead. Eventually, he caught me staring in his direction. I was relieved when he waved his notepad, then leaned towards me pointing a pen, rather than his revolver.

"You're awake?"

"How long was I out?"

"Not long. An hour or so. You'll be fine. You're Jeffrey Hanson, right?"

"No, Jeff is my dad."

"We ran your plates." He checked his notes. "Jeffery Mark Hanson."

"I guess I screwed up, huh?"

"You were doing over 50 through two red lights. Drunk. No license."

"In that case," I sighed, "I'm John Doe."

"You're not John Doe. He's in surgery. What's your name?"

A young nurse appeared. She checked my pulse and eyes, then asked a few questions. I grinned at the Sheriff, then gave her my name and address so that she could complete my intake. She kept smiling. Maybe it was a bit of residual shock from the morning's ordeal, but while giving her my phone number, I almost added that she did not have to worry about HIPAA... that I would be flattered if she'd keep that number for personal use.

"Mark, you'll be fine," she smiled, patting my arm. "The drugs and drip have worked their magic. You'll be out of here in good order in no time."

"Wonderful." She really did have a nice smile. "Ma'am, it really has been a pleasure. You have a wonderful bedside manner." I nodded at the window. "Him, not so much."

She laughed. She checked the IV, then made a few more notations on my chart.

"You're from Denver," she said. "You should know better. Lots of water. Always. No alcohol this high on an empty stomach." She shook her head. "No mountain driving under the influence."

She glanced at the Sheriff, then corrected herself.

"No mountain driving... when you're sick."

"So what's going on?" I asked. "What about the other guy?"

She met my eyes and shook her head, ever-so-slightly, yes.

"Can I use the bathroom? How soon can I check out?"

"Hold on, tiger," she smiled. "I've got to watch what I say, but yes, you can use the bathroom. Sheriff, do you want to help him... or should I?"

I raised my hand. "I'm okay for now. I was just wondering for later."

She finished her charting, adjusted the IV, then promised she'd be back to unleash me in ten minutes when the bag was dry. That would be a good time to use the bathroom.

I watched her leave, thankful that she'd been so calm. She had to know about the plane. I wished she'd been able to tell me something. I closed my eyes for a moment and searched my gut to see if I was steady.

"Seriously," I said, opening my eyes to the sheriff. "Why are you here? Am I under arrest?"

"Right now, no. Probably never. But we've got a lot of questions. You ready to talk?"

"I've got plenty of questions myself."

"Yours will have to wait. We can't say a thing right now except that you're a witness and a participant in something big enough to draw agents and big shots from around the country. Feds, engineers, Denver CSI, Homeland Security. You name it, they're all on the way. Driving faster than you. But sober. Some in helicopters. All with lots of questions."

"I don't know anything. What do you know?"

"My questions first."

"Can you at least tell me if the guy I brought down is going to be okay? Do you know who he is?"

"Can't say."

"Not fair. You're killing me."

"Get used to it."

SUNDAY NEWS

They kept me in the hospital and away from the media for as long as they could. Officially, that was "overnight for observation," which actually amounted to another 24 hours of off-and-on interrogations. Thankfully, between sessions they let me nap and eat pretty well, and then eventually turn on the television. In short order, I began learning from the cable networks where me and my guy fit into the nightmare playing out in Los Angeles, Chicago, and, damn it, again in New York.

Not to mention the four planes that had been dropped in Europe.

Plus a ninth in the Mediterranean Sea off the coast of Israel.

Scenes of carnage and grief flowed non-stop on every channel.

American planes had been destroyed strategically and simultaneously in four scattered regions around the country. Speculation and fear ran amok as to how such an attack was possible in an age of multi-billion dollar security. Judging from numerous high-level interviews and press conferences, TSA and Homeland Security were in the midst of a meltdown. Borders were closed and nobody knew anything. Or at least nobody was saying. Air travel was locked down at virtually every non-military airport in the world.

A weeping Chicago woman who'd nearly been hit by a falling briefcase declared during her interview: "There was no place to hide from the falling skies."

Within an hour, the essence of her phrase had morphed and taken on an authoritative edge. Aggressive journalists at other crash sites began probing their witnesses for graphic recollections from their own experiences with the "falling skies" of that deadly day.

By twilight, "The Day of the Falling Skies" and "The Falling Skies Massacre" had become the universal handles for the events, and those coordinated savage attacks were certain to be remembered as such in all future histories— if any such books would ever be written again.

That night the President aired a brief statement from an undisclosed location. He expressed deep grief and impassioned moral outrage. Pending the results of intelligence reports, a fuller update and statement from the White House was promised for sometime within the next 24 hours.

Hundreds of millions of people around the globe were frightened. Families and friends grieved. Politicians screamed for action. Someone needed to pay, and judging by many of the man-on-the-street live reactions, it almost didn't seem to matter who.

According to a sidebar story, participation in Palm Sunday worship services around the world hit an all-time low. Opinions varied as to whether the faithful were staying home glued to the news, or because they were afraid to gather in public venues. Or both.

I sat in my bed, half-glad they held me on lockdown. I wanted to get my bearings. Rumors of me and my stranger from beneath the snow were leaking all over the place. Hundreds of careers in politics and media were going to be made or trashed within the next 30 days, and I didn't want to be anyone's pawn. The world wanted to know who this guy was, and the media wanted to tell them. Hints that me and my guy were the only bright spots in this real-time global nightmare made me queasy. They wanted our story.

Now.

Knowing what I'd eventually be facing when I walked out their door, the hospital sent me a psychologist.

They also sent a lawyer, a case manager, and a chaplain. In that order. Each left a card, along with a few suggestions. I let the chaplain pray, because he seemed to need that.

All morning the second day, I watched through my window. A pool of sharks circled below, growing in size by the hour. Mobile media rigs flowed in from every direction.

Law enforcement types rallied in force, roping off and commandeering an entire half of the parking lot. Television crews and production trucks from Denver docked first, establishing camps in all the best locations. Late arrivals from national teams and other states lined the driveway, then stretched beyond the parking lot out onto Highway 9, which made for chaos because of the narrow shoulders and frozen slush.

I recognized a couple of the closest talking heads from Denver stations, and I was not surprised to see who landed the best berth on the lot: Saundra Paige, from Channel 5's "High-5-at-Five" News.

Her team must have been the first to arrive because their satellite truck and equipment sprawled nearly all the way to the hospital's front door. They held court over twice the space allotted to any of the other stations. Saundra swayed sweet and lovely as always. Perfect face, perfect lips, perfectly highlighted hair. Perfect everything. The princess wore a sweeping blue wool cape today, tailored to accentuate her perfectly adorable figure.

She directed her teams with a commanding regal flair, swinging arms for lighting and sound, elevating beauty and order from the pandemonium below. And only thirty-something.

With a flick of her wrist, she drew a wiry intern to her side. She consulted the cell phone in her left hand, passed him a few bills, then sent him spinning off in the direction of a long shivering line.

A local concessions entrepreneur had somehow finagled a spot for his 4x dually and trailer. A long stream of over-dressed personalities and under-dressed crews snaked through twenty-five feet of melting parking slop, all waiting their turns to be watered and fed.

A crew from Santa Fe with a stunning desert mural on their van was broadcasting from the gas station across the street. Another live remote with a Moab Arch decal pulled to a stop, apparently fresh from the Salt Lake City Trail. Small teams fluttered in and out like bees, gathering crash debris footage and interviews from around the valley, all to be edited and uplinked from the media hub and improvised broadcast center below.

Saundra disappeared, and I began to lose interest.

A dirty city truck bellowed onto the scene with a set of gray porta-potties. Two gorillas jumped out to stomp and beat their chests. They gruffly wrestled to offload their crude essentials, then lined them up like personal monuments alongside the hospital drive.

They strutted and swore, daring anyone to actually approach. I shuddered, then turned from the window, clicked off the television and tried to take a nap.

"He wants to see you."

"Who is it this time?"

I'd grown fond of my keeper. His name was Mr. Deputy Sheriff, and he had all the endearing personality traits of his black-holstered sidearm.

"The guy from the plane."

I feigned shock. "He's alive?"

Of course I knew he was alive. Five billion people knew. It was now everywhere on the news, even though they'd not yet officially released his name. Passenger lists and body identifications and family notifications were all going terribly slow. Everything was being double and triple checked for accuracy.

The terrorists had been strategic with their targets. The Denver-bound Airbus dropped nearly 300 passengers from high above the Rockies. It would be weeks, if ever, before families and communities would find resolution. Investigators would be spread thin. Fresh stories would churn in the news cycle for months. The shock, distress and fear would stir again each time a piece of debris or clothing—or bone—popped through the melting snow in a remote canyon... or in some vacationer's backyard.

"Don't screw with me," Sheriff frowned. "You know he's alive. This is serious."

"Of course it's serious. Everything is serious." I hadn't meant to be so ironic. My reply was on reflex. In truth, I was stunned to imagine seeing the man from the tree. After a deep breath, I restarted in a more civil tone.

"He's talking?"

"Not really. He refuses to answer any of the questions that count. He says he wants to meet with you... first. Before he'll talk to anyone else."

"Like I said, I don't even know the guy."

"Maybe you do, maybe you don't."

"I think," I sighed, "I would know if I knew him."

"Maybe not. Not with his face in shreds. But maybe if he was strutting around on television in a suit you, then would might recognize him."

I sat up.

"Who is this guy? He's famous? He's on television?"

"Let's just say... if he fully recovers, then this little episode will not hurt his ratings any in the days to come."

Hmm. "He can talk, but only to me? Why me?"

"Ask him."

ALONE WITH FREAK

5

I couldn't believe it when the escort team showed up with a wheelchair. My strength had fully returned, and I was feeling completely myself. Other than the surreal fog that hung over everything that had just happened to me—and to planet Earth—I was fine.

An entourage of jacket-and-ties, along with a couple of sets of pale blue scrubs, together forced me to sit and ride. When I threatened to sue, the oldest nurse smiled, "My husband's a lawyer." She caught herself in an administrator's glare, then promptly dropped her gaze.

Flanked and outnumbered, I changed floors. We turned a few corners, then slowed to a halt outside a conference room door. Through the glass panes beside the entrance, I caught a flurry of activity and a menagerie of medical paraphernalia that, like me, must have been wheeled in from obscure hideaways from around the building. I didn't notice any TV's.

"As you can imagine," said one the starchiest of the suits, "we'll be recording everything. In fairness, my disclosure needs to be on the record."

"No problem," I nodded. "Just send me a copy on DVD. I could use something new for next weekend. I'm behind on my cable payments, and they've been threatening to cut me off."

"We've already informed the other patient of the same. Knowing our position, he still demands to speak with you. Alone." He shook his head. "We're having a hard time assessing the extent of his psychological trauma and brain damage."

"What's his name? What should I call him?"

"See what he says. We know his name, but he refuses to confirm or deny. He says nothing. Your conversation will hopefully fill in some gaps. As I mentioned, we're still running a battery of neurological exams." They pushed me through the door. "Again, as said, we'll be recording."

I don't know what I expected.

His face was almost entirely hidden beneath a mask of gauze. He was hooked to several machines and two drips. As I stepped out from my wheelchair and approached his bed, the medical staff quickly collected stainless steel trays and odds and ends and moved as far away as space allowed. A pair of suits stepped briskly from the room, and one hit the record button on a tiny camera mounted on the arm of a swinging lamp. The remaining ten or so observers retreated to various nooks and equipment gaps as best they could.

Apparently we were now alone.

I stood a moment, trying to inventory the damage. White wrappings covered most of John Doe's head, presumably to protect against infection and to hold the loose flesh in place. His nose was a bump beneath the wrap, and he'd only been left small slits for eyes. His mouth and chin were exposed and intact, though stained yellow and pink.

As best I could tell, all his parts were in about the right places. I stepped closer, trying confirm what I could about his eyes... if they were really there, and if so, whether they could focus through all that wrapped gauze and swelling. I counted. Yes. Two dark eyes. Yes, both open. Both tracking... presumably in sufficient working order.

"Hello, " I said at last. I waited. "Glad you made it. Sorry about your face. You okay?"

For maybe the longest minute of my life, I watched for even a tick. At last, he broke the silence with a whisper.

"Come closer.... As close as you can."

What could I do? I stepped forward and leaned until my ear was only inches from his mouth. I could smell the ointments. Could almost taste the gauze. And maybe some fermenting blood.

"Thank you," he said, his voice so faint I could hardly hear. Another long pause. "God has chosen well."

I blinked. I waited some more, now understanding the concern of the suit-and-scrubs about the possibility of brain damage. Nothing else for a while, so I eventually straightened, my spine feeling stiffer than after I'd dragged him from his icy grave.

"More..." he whispered.

Reluctantly, I leaned over once again.

"No accidents." His voice was lower, raspier this time. Then a whole lot more nothing.

I glanced towards the somber team protecting the windows and walls, then shrugged. There wasn't any more that I could read on their faces than from his, so I turned and dropped my head and stared again into his eyes, barely inches from mine. The lights were on. Somebody pretended to be home. But how could he, of all people in the world, dare to mutter, "No accidents"? I decided to ask.

I moved my lips to the vicinity of his ear.

"Dude," I whispered back, "you were thrown from a plane two miles above the Rocky Mountains... without a parachute. You landed at terminal velocity in a pine tree in a stranger's backyard. Was that your plan?"

Quietly, he chuckled.

"I'm glad," I grinned, "you've still got your sense of humor. Does it hurt to talk?"

"Only when I laugh," he whispered.

"Are you laughing a lot these days?"

"That was the first time." The right corner of his mouth twitched. I caught a little sparkle in his eyes. "God is good. He's blocking the pain."

"Right. The doctors are good, too." I pointed to one of the drips. "That one says, 'Morphine.'"

"Good enough. Both are true." He studied me for a moment. "I'm supposed to tell you something. I'm not sure why...."

"And?"

"No accidents."

I glanced over my shoulder. The huddle of scrubs leaned my way. I shook my head.

"Mister, you already said that. You're not making sense. You've had a bad accident...."

"Okay," his voice gained strength. "Accidents can happen. At least from one perspective. Not the big stuff, though. Not like you think."

"What do you mean?"

"Things may seem random, but there are no true accidents.... not when properly understood."

I might have winced.

"What's wrong?" he asked. "You okay?"

"Am I okay? Bud, have you seen a mirror lately?" I grinned. "No, I'm okay."

"Then why did you jerk your head like that?"

"I didn't jerk. I winced."

"Okay. And...."

"I've kinda heard the saying before. Except what I got was the opposite version. You say there are no accidents. The way I was taught—when properly understood—there are no...." I hesitated.

For some reason, my mouth was too dry to finish. Probably all of the whispering. I licked my lips and swallowed. "There are no... *miracles.*"

Behind me, a cell phone started playing from somebody's pocket. An absurd show tune. A quick fumble, a click, then silence. It had to have been a nurse. No respectable doctor or any government dark suit would be carrying anything from *Mikado* in their pants. I was tempted to peek.

My guy moved his head, ever so slightly, drawing me back down close enough to receive yet another secret.

"You were taught wrong. Look at me. A miracle."

I stretched my back and gave him a thorough once over. I decided to withhold my final verdict on miracles pending more data. I did notice for the first time his hand. No wounds or scratches. It rested on his chest, sporting an oversized gold ring. I leaned tight.

"You married? Are you expecting your wife soon?"

"I'm not sure."

"You're not sure if you're married?"

He snorted, lightly. It was a relief to know that under all that gauze, at least his nose still worked.

"My wife and kids are in California. With the airlines down, that'd be a long drive."

"It's a long drive even when the planes are flying. Do they know if you survived?"

"I suspect the authorities called them."

"You haven't called them yourself? Who are you, anyway?"

"You don't know?"

"I've got no idea who you are. I'm not sure if *you* even know. They've complained," I gestured over my shoulder, "you've been pretty tight lipped." I smiled. "They think you've got brain damage. By the way, do I really have to keep leaning over like this? My back is killing me."

He laughed again, less softly. He invited me to pull up a chair. After I'd settled, he continued.

"My brain is fine. I'm from the Bay area. I was flying out of San Francisco, headed to Chicago for a special conference. Because of all the late spring snow in Chicago, I was rerouted. My new flight gave me a connection in Denver. I wasn't even supposed to be on that plane. I'm supposed to be in Chicago right now... presenting to a national audience."

"A national audience? What kind of business are you in?"

"It's a religious conference. For Palm Sunday. I'm a preacher. I was invited to speak at a major summit, a gathering called to discuss the End Times. The end of the world."

I knew what the End Times were.

"There is not," he added, "a lot of sand left in the hourglass."

"Right."

I'd read the first two books of the *Left Behind* series on a $50 bet after a couple of beers at a sports bar. Not only that, I'd also seen Nicholas Cage play the idiot pilot during a blind date with my sister's cute-but-silly Christian best friend. I knew all about the apocalypse, inside and out. Now I was starting to understand the kind of kook I was dealing with. A guy who speaks at conferences about Grim Reapers. A fan of mayhem and the nonsense of the End of Days.

"So," I asked, "do you think your pilot was raptured?"

"Of course not!"

"Good," I said, genuinely thankful. "Because the whole absurd idea of someone just leaving a plane at cruising altitude...."

He laughed, waiting a moment for me to catch the irony. Then he leaned a few inches towards me, as if to spill a deadly global scoop.

"There is much we must do, and not much time. Like it or not, a lot has fallen to me. And to you. We've been set apart. We're going to be very busy between now and Armageddon."

Hmm.

"A national conference, eh? What did you say your name was?"

"Bill Jacobs. I have a church and television ministry near San Francisco."

"Is your show the one they call, 'The Final Hour'?"

"Correct. You've seen it?"

"Never."

"Oh."

"I've only heard about you and your show through the jokes they tell on late night television. No offense."

"None taken. The jokes are good for our ratings. In the media, there's no such thing as bad publicity."

"Kinda ironic, though, a weekly show called 'The Last Hour.' Is your contract by the season, or by the episode?"

He laughed again, a bit too hardy. I started to worry about his stitches. "Actually, we have a number of contracts. Some are with churches, some are with local stations. Some are with the networks." He studied my face. "Some are by the event... others are by the year."

"Big business."

"Very."

"Well, congratulations. Business is going to be booming."

"We'll see. I'm still trying to figure this all out. I've been lying here the past 24 hours doing a lot of praying. A lot of listening."

"Besides all of the doctor-and-nurse gossip, what have you been hearing?"

"God told me that I had fallen."

Hmm. A genius.

"And God also told me that He would raise me up again."

"No broken legs, huh?"

He studied me for closely.

"I've got a bad hip. It hurts. But as I said, God is working on the pain. God always takes care of me." He grinned. "And, as *you* say, the medications help. I landed feet first, and I jammed it pretty hard."

"I should think. Not to worry, though. I heard that God is going to raise you up. He must really love you.'"

"He does. And He loves you, too."

"Right." I shifted a few inches away from his bed rail.

The "God loves you" pitch always drives me a little crazy. I'd never met a television preacher before. Sometimes I'd see them on TV, and on each occasion, I'd debated with them, the way I did with the dead philosophers I'd read in college. I should have felt more sympathy for this guy after what he'd been through. Instead, I found myself reacting to him as if he were on my television screen, strutting in his flashy suit rather than stiff under a sheet in a hospital gown.

"You doubt?" He sounded surprised. Disappointed.

"Sure," I said, starting to tremble. "God loves you. He saved you. Here you are, Bill, safe and sound. The other 2,000 people who didn't walk away yesterday... maybe God loves them... not so much?"

It was Bill's turn to wince.

"You think," he said at last, "that you mock me." His voice dropped low, almost angry. "But you mock yourself. And you mock the Lord. I see it now. You've got a spiritual attachment." He dug into me with his eyes. "At least one Dark Rider, maybe more. I see a spirit of...."

"Stop it." I jerked back. "I don't believe in God. And I certainly don't believe in mumbo-jumbo like 'Riders' and 'spiritual attachments.' Whatever the heck they are." I shook my head. "No. Don't tell me. I don't even want to know."

He closed his eyes. A siren rose and fell outside, coming to a stop by the ER entrance. The airlines might be down, but not the gondolas. Probably another broken leg shuttled in from the slopes.

"God knows," he said, raising two fingers, "what he is doing. He chose you for a reason, just as He chose me. You need to wrap your head around this. Like it or not, you have become a player in something very big. As big as it gets."

"Hey, friend, you seem like an interesting guy. Let's do coffee and swap a few memories about this someday when you're feeling better." I started to get up to leave.

"Stop it." The edge in his voice was suddenly commanding. "You need to quit thinking you had a choice in this. You need to stop thinking like you can simply walk away from the Creator of the Universe and do whatever you want."

I glared back. I leaned so close that I could again smell his bandages and blood.

"Do you really presume to know what I am thinking?"

"What if I do?"

We've all got our red buttons, and this pompous charlatan with his God-loves-you clichés and his know-it-all attitudes had just slapped his palm hard on one of my hottest.

"What am I thinking now?" I dared.

He dared me back with a stare.

Of all the people in the world to survive… a television preacher! I heard a doctor shuffling nervously by the window. From the corner of my eye, I caught an agent in the midst of a frantic scribble.

The Reverend Bill Jacobs met my eyes and burrowed. I refused to turn or blink.

Who was this guy? A fruitcake… or merely a self-righteous jerk? My focus blurred, but I drilled back with all I could muster. My rage sharpened. I'd give him plenty to read.

And then I remembered. I'd seen Jacobs once before, on his show. He'd been peddling his End Times flip chart, actually looking giddy as he explained all the sickening ways he predicted people to die. He must have been brain damaged long before he met the Rockies face-to-face.

Suddenly, Jacobs turned to the empty side of his bed. And chuckled.

I snatched a quick blink. Angry, but relieved.

"You lose." I shook my head. "You claimed that you could read my mind. And then you laughed. If you knew what I was thinking, you certainly would not have found it funny. You're a fake. No offense, preacher."

"None taken, sinner. Now I know."

"What?"

"This was a test. We passed. You'll make a perfect witness. In your own way, you're as volatile and stubborn as I am. God is more clever than people imagine."

"You just made it about God again. You're cheating. You never said what I was thinking."

"I think... that you were thinking that I landed on my head."

"And?"

"Brain damage. You were thinking that I must have jarred a screw loose. And... and you were feeling that I should have died. It should have been someone else who survived."

"Good guess." I straightened.

"For the last time, Mark. No brain injuries."

"Look," I said. "Maybe no brain damage. Maybe God has a plan, or maybe you're just the luckiest man alive. Either way, it was a freak deal." I patted his hand. "You can be a God freak on a freak'n God mission if you want, but count me out. I'm not a guy to save the whales... let alone the world."

Again I waited for a reply, starting to suspect that maybe his long pauses weren't just about exhaustion. Finally, I started to leave.

"*Freak.*" He said it gently, testing the ring of it. "I like that. A God freak.... the Freak Fall Miracle survivor." The little snatches of his face not in gauze seemed happy. "Mark, like I said, God knew what He was doing when He threw us together."

"I'm glad, Reverend Jacobs, that you and God are on such good terms. Gotta confess, though, God and me... not so much."

"Yes, Mark, I can see that."

It suddenly registered that he was using my name.

"How do you know my name? We've never met. Did they tell you...."

"No. They never said."

"Well, don't give me that line that I just look like a Mark."

More of the waiting game. When he answered, his voice floated as softly as when I'd first walked in.

"Mark," he whispered, forcing me to again lean close. "Do you see anything..." he motioned with a finger, "over there? Perhaps something shimmering?"

"Your IV bag?"

"No, more of a God thing." His voice shifted. "Maybe you'll understand later. Then let's call the *Mark* guess a lucky accident."

"Right. From 20,000 feet, Mr. Lucky walks. Thousands of names, and he nails mine in one guess. What are the odds? No doubt... I've really met the luckiest man alive."

He closed his eyes. "Maybe I am getting tired. You're right, it's been an ordeal." His eyes opened, sad. "The folks along the wall are not quite done with me yet, and I'm not up for any more hostility right now." He settled his hand back upon his chest. "What's next for you, Mark?"

The room fell utterly silent, save for the hum and beep of a nearby monitor.

I wondered how messed up the poor guy truly might be. My sympathy must have showed, because he met my concern with a reply.

"I'm not as messed up as you might think."

"Preacher, you're messing with my head. How am I supposed to know what I'm going to do next? I came up to the mountains to relax. I'm not the one who hears from God. I didn't ask for the media to gather outside my window. I didn't ask for any of this. Bill...."

"Freak. You need to call me *Freak*. The name is going to stick. I'm taking it with me to the press conference and interviews when I walk out of here tomorrow evening."

"Freak," I said, testing the sound of it myself. "You're discharging yourself out of the hospital like this? I don't know what to say. I guess we're back to that whole landing-on-your-head business?"

"Stop it. You know I didn't land on my head. I crashed through a hundred feet of pine boughs heavy with snow. I rolled through the branches and hit deep snow, feet first, then slid down a sharp angle that flattened to where you could dig me out. It's a miracle that I was wearing a heavy parka, a miracle that I hit in the exact right place in the exact right tree, a miracle that you pulled me out in time."

"Or luck?"

"Not luck. Miracle."

"And you know this because....?"

"The angels told me." He studied my blank stare. "Two angels were with me, laughing and talking and singing the whole way down. Telling me to trust. After I landed, I distinctly remember beginning to panic... when the tunnel above me started to collapse. The little air passage began to close, and I wanted to scream for help. I could barely move a finger in that frozen cocoon, and I was running out of air. And then the angel of the Lord commanded, 'Relax. Save your oxygen. Mark is on the way.'"

Again, I was speechless.

"And," he finished firmly, "you know darn well that it was only by the strength of those angels that you were able to dig me out and haul me here in time."

"Angels?"

"Of course. One of them is here right now." He nodded to the empty side of his bed.

Like an idiot, I looked.

He turned his gaze to the suits and scrubs, who shifted nervously, pretending not to be straining to catch every word. "I'm going to tell them everything I know soon enough. Not that any of them will believe. It's all on video anyway." He nodded towards the tiny camera. "First, though, I needed to hear from God and to collect myself in order to get a few things straight."

"You really think you hear from God?"

"That's what drives me. Every day. It is critical that I hear and boldly obey. Let the chips fall. And who or what is it that drives you, Mark?" He studied me for a moment. "Let's try again. Mark... what are your plans?"

It was my turn to close my eyes and wait. I replayed what I could of the past conversation, breathing slow and deep, trying to sort it out. Feeling way in over my head. A bit like I was under the snow, my air passage collapsing, hoping for someone to dig me out. This was all too unreal.

I opened my eyes, glancing to where he said the angel stood.

I saw nothing.

But the hair on my arm tingled all the same.

"I've got no idea," I said, brushing my sleeve. "I don't know what I'm going to do. I've got a few more days of vacation. Then I suppose I'll head back to Denver to finish the semester. I'm a teacher."

"You should have given this more thought by now." He quivered, then sank back. "The media is going to tear you apart. You'll need some help with this."

"What about you, what's God telling you to do? There's no way the hospital is going to discharge you in this condition."

"By tomorrow afternoon, I will no longer be like this. In the morning, I'll be healed."

Hmm. I could breathe again. It got a lot easier when he was crazy.

"Listen... I, ah...."

"Freak. You've got to start calling me Freak. It'll help the cause immensely."

"Right." I leaned away. "Freak, I don't think that I can commit to your cause. I've got a pleasant little life, and I'm eager to get back to the sanity and safety of what I know. The good life. You and your supposed mission are way too far out there for me."

"My mission? Haven't you been listening? *Our* mission."

"Look, Freak. Right now you're the most amazing person in the world. Everybody's going to want to hear what you have to say. You don't need me. I'm only a run-of-the-mill school teacher. I'm ready to go home. In a few days, I've got to be ready to give a lecture about Hamlet and start grading essays. Back to the real world for me."

"Call in sick. Quit your job. It doesn't matter. That job is not your future." He paused. "I am."

"Right."

"Seriously. Life as you've known it is over. What do you suppose is going to happen when you step out that door later today?"

I hesitated.

"Do this. Tell these folks," he nodded to the wall, "tell the guy in the black tie that you want them to put you up in a nice secured hotel room for a few days while you try to deal with the media frenzy and sort things out. Tell them you've got some PTS, and you're afraid you'll do or say something stupid."

"Actually, that's probably true." I smiled. "But I have a cabin. I don't need a hotel room. Besides, long about now, there's probably not a room left anywhere in Summit County."

"They'll find you something. The hotel room won't be only for you... it's for both of us. Get the room today, and I'll join you tomorrow night. If you change your mind, check out early and leave me the keys."

I considered.

"Mark, what do you have to lose?"

"Should I ask for room service?"

"Heck yes! Milk this. Don't miss out... this is a chance of a lifetime. Run up a huge tab. Live like a king. Have some fun with it."

Hmm. Now he was finally making sense. For the first time, Freak was talking my kind of language.

"Who," he asked, "should be the reporter to get the scoop on my story? I don't know the local stations. Pick one, and they'll get my first interview, later today. An exclusive. The rest of them will have to wait until I officially come out at tomorrow's press conference."

He seemed to thoroughly believe what he was saying. He really thought he was going to be healed.

I shrugged. The lovely Saundra Paige came to mind.

"We've got a Denver station that gets a lot of respect, and they're considered a stellar network affiliate. Channel 5."

"Good." He raised his head a few inches.

"Folks," he said, addressing the windows and walls, his voice surprisingly strong. "I am all yours for the next hour. I'm going to answer all of your questions as best I can. Nothing but the truth, so help me God. And then, in exchange, I want you to arrange an interview with Denver's Channel 5 News."

Several suits glanced at each other, nervously wondering who would take the lead.

"Folks," his voice now commanding, "let's shoot for a live interview in time for tonight's Channel 5 News. Everybody is dying to know the meaning and the far-reaching implications of the Falling Skies Massacre. Let's not keep the world waiting any longer."

THE INTERVIEW

How Freak got everything he wanted so quickly, I'll never know. Within a few hours, I found myself in a massive Breckenridge townhouse unit seven miles up the mountain from Frisco. I stood in the vaulted great room, two bags of new, donated sportswear in hand, staring out through a twenty-foot glass wall at a breathtaking view of a dozen of the finest ski runs in Colorado. The executive condo sported a classic five star floor plan, done in rustic pine with an open loft, two bedrooms up and two more down, three bathrooms, a game room, a central living room, two fireplaces, a kitchen, and a fully stocked bar.

I soon found myself nestled under a wool blanket with a bottle of sweet Riesling on a tremendous overstuffed leather sectional couch. Placated and fascinated, I watched Freak playfully bantering with Saundra Paige on High-5-at Five News.

My own press conference was a madhouse blur. A huge white carnival tent had been trucked down from the festival up in Breckenridge, complete with sandbag weights, folding chairs, generators, and several commercial grade propane heaters. The hospital's case manager scrounged up an impressive selection of snazzy sportswear and ball caps for me to choose from, all with conspicuous local and national brand logos. They led me out the front door and down through a roped corridor to the media circus tent in the parking lot, my good friend Deputy Sheriff locked on one elbow, a federal agent with stale breath guiding my other.

A gray coiffed spokesperson representing the hospital raised his hand to open the festivities. He read a prepared press release that was also now available on the clinic's web site, and then briskly recited a standard set of procedural protocols. He promised to keep the session short, then abruptly threw me to the sharks.

I read an informative five-paragraph statement.

Also now available on the hospital's web site.

Several of us had collaborated on the piece an hour prior. I thought it was pretty good, maybe a B+. It cast the hospital in a favorable light, celebrated that the victim would probably survive, and it made me out to be a bit of a minor hero.

Standing there before all those cameras, all of those intense engineer nerds and technical directors, and a handful of gorgeously manicured talking heads, I held my own. A few years of public speaking in front of six rows of high school jocks, cheerleaders and dope heads finally paid off. The press folks were taking notes, wagging their heads, and collecting non-stop images from every angle.

Near the end of my prepared statement, we were interrupted briefly by one of the many helicopters to come and go in the valley over the next few days. In the deep bowl of the Summit County central valley, the acoustical droning and sub-tonal impact of these flights was significantly unsettling. This one swooped over low, with a rapid thumpf-sha-thumpf-sha, indicating a small traffic-news copter from one of the Denver stations. The military cargo and utility helicopters from Fort Carson produced a much deeper thump-reverb, such that I'd often find myself stopping whatever I was doing in order to absorb and manage their ominous passing.

The news chopper swept around above the tent twice, then quickly headed off towards the little airport outside of town.

My summary statement paragraph was unembellished, providing mostly repeats from my previous interviews with the agents and staff behind me. I concluded my report with the most essential and personal of all details: I was a nobody. I really didn't know anything. Questions? Let the shouting and arm thrusting begin.

Some answers required only simple reworkings of statements I'd already made. Yes, I actually did see the explosion, and yes, I did see the body hit... or at least, I saw it disappear into the trees a short distance up the mountain behind my deck.

Other questions were inappropriate, like whether or not I had any theories as to why terrorists would do such a thing. They must have mistaken me for someone else: Dudes, I reminded them, I'm nobody. I don't know anything. I was just sitting on my deck reading a book.

Many of the questions were garbled and indecipherable. I focused as best I could on the handful of questions that I felt comfortable with. As instructed by my coaches beforehand, whenever I needed to, I blamed the PTS of the explosion and carnage and the exhaustion of digging and dragging him out. I also improvised at one point that the trauma of this press conference was alone sufficient explanation for any notable lapses in my coherence. Many of them seemed delighted by my confession; they seemed flattered to imagine themselves so intimidating.

In contrast to most such nonsense, the three questions from forward-leaning Miss Paige were articulate, to the point, and got the best answers I could summon... after I'd finally been able to clear my throat.

Yes, I had spoken today with the survivor. Yes, the Reverend Bill Jacobs was now answering to the name, "Freak." No, I didn't know whether or not his survival of the Falling Skies Massacre should be called a miracle. It might have been luck.

Saundra seemed a little disappointed.

She smiled a thank you, then relinquished the floor to the orcish others. To the brutish carnivores and the plastic bobble heads of the competing venues.

A couple hours later, there Saundra was again, relaxed, smooth, beautiful, chatting it up with a good-natured mummy on the five o'clock news.

The room where Freak and I first met had been transformed into a television studio of sorts, complete with ferns, balanced lighting, and a glass table with two bottled waters and a potted floral arrangement in reds, whites, and blues.

The effect was surreal. The world in chaos, and Saundra smiling with an end-times preacher nodding a head swathed in brilliant white gauze. The horror of airplane debris and bodies plummeting into the valley yesterday around my back deck. And then one day later, me sipping expensive wine as vacationers zipped up Peak 6 on the Kensho SuperChair lift barely beyond the glass plates of my breathtaking new view.

The happy guest on Channel 5 News was down to one IV bag, and despite the facial shroud, he projected the epitome of abundant life. His bed had been lowered and adjusted into a recliner mode; his hospital bed sheet had been swapped out for a cozy lap comforter, complete with a resort name and local ski scene prominently displayed.

Saundra was in high form. Her pacing and progression of questions was perfect, laced with her girl-next-door charm... on a network feed beaming live, planet-wide, to an audience of several hundred million.

"Well," laughed Freak, "as the joke goes, it's not the long fall... it's the sudden stop at the end that will get you."

"And...?" smiled Saundra.

"God spared me the sudden stop at the end. He caught me in His arms."

"His arms?"

"An enormous evergreen... perfectly positioned, with drooping flexible boughs thick with needles and padded with mounds of freshly fallen snow."

"You did pass through the tree and hit the ground though, eventually?"

"Not exactly. From those branches that slowed my fall and turned me vertical, I was then released into deep snow, fluffy on top, then increasingly hard and packed after several feet down. Also, it was almost as if I was dropped feet first onto the top of a children's playground slider. Not at all like striking a flat surface."

He raised his hand. "Picture my right hand up here as the spot where I entered the snow." He tipped his elbow out and placed his left hand in his raised palm. "The angle was perfect, steep at the top," he slid his hand down to his elbow. "I plowed through deep snow like I was slipping down a child's slider until I finally slowed to a complete halt."

"So, you're saying that there was no sudden stop at the end."

"Exactly."

"As you know," smiled Saundra, "the eyes of the world are upon you. You truly are an amazing story."

"The story," quipped Freak, "is God." He nodded and continued, his voice stronger, his eyes and mouth beneath the wrappings more expressive than I remembered from that afternoon.

"I am just one of God's endless miracles. Every day, every hour. Me... a miracle. The teacher who found me near his cabin... a miracle." I winced. "And you, Ms. Paige."

I swear, I saw a little wink through all of that gauze.

Then, turning to the camera, he blithely declared to the world. "God's miracles are for everyone. If you are watching, God's miracles are for you, too. Know this: the cliché is reliable. Miracles never cease."

Saundra laughed. No condescension. Pure childlike delight.

"Thank you, Reverend Jacobs, for reminding us. Tonight, in the aftermath of the Falling Skies Massacre, there are millions of people around the globe who need this kind of encouragement."

"Yes. We must not lose hope."

"Maybe now," Saundra nodded off camera, "I think it would be a good time to roll a short clip."

The video opened with me. I was practically falling out of the SUV, on national television, fumbling to lift the back lid of my vehicle, blubbering, shouting, not making a lot of sense. She must have been up in Breckenridge covering the Winter Festival—she must have charged straight down to the hospital when she saw the jet explosion above the valley. Medical staff were everywhere, pulling me aside, hauling out a gurney, transferring him, then rushing him inside. Saundra provided a scripted voice over:

"At first, nobody had any idea who you were, or that you'd fallen from the plane. Thank God Mark Hanson found you so quickly and got you here to the Frisco Trauma Center in time."

"Yes, thank God for everything."

Hmm. Yes, thank God Saundra chose to cut the clip before the part where I bent over and started to puke.

"Were you conscious at this time? Do you remember being admitted to the hospital?"

"No, thank God. The Lord allowed me to black out for the last part of my ordeal. I remember no pain from the facial injuries."

"So... you clearly believe that God was with you throughout this entire miracle."

The screen filled with a file photo of Pastor Bill Jacobs, a vibrant man, mid-40's, speaking to a vast audience from an elevated stage loaded with props and lush California foliage.

Then back to a tight live shot of Saundra's face. "You keep coming back to God whenever you discuss what happened."

"Yes, I keep returning to God for everything. Where else would you go in times like these?"

"Some of our viewers may have heard of you, or even watched you on television before. Your San Francisco-based ministry, the 'Bill Jacob's Final Hour,' is broadcasted in many of the biggest markets in the nation."

"Thanks for the plug." As he nodded, the screen went to a split image, a tight live shot of his swaying mummy head on the left, a flattering magazine cover photo of the preacher to the right.

"We know you've been through a lot, a unique horror beyond imagination."

"Actually, it wasn't so bad," he chuckled. "Not that I'd want to do it again anytime soon."

Saundra shook her head and grinned. "Let's roll our second clip."

Suddenly, I was looking at my cabin's back deck. My open novel, face down, and a few empty beer bottles, all still on the table. Then a slow pan up my deep snow trail to and from the pines. I couldn't spot any yellow crime scene tape. She must have beaten the feds to the site. Then a zoom on the dark spills of blood where I'd checked him for breathing and pulse.

How did she get this footage? I closed my eyes and waited a moment for a shudder of remembered exhaustion and nausea to pass.

"You probably don't recall any of this, but here we see the cabin deck and the national forest area where you were rescued."

"Correct. I don't remember seeing any of this. I only had a vague sense of what was happening at this point. I was slipping in and out of awareness from the time I hit until later in the hospital."

"Here we see the path where Mark Hanson snowshoed in to save you, and where he later dragged you back out."

The cameraman must have been wearing snowshoes himself to follow my tracks through such deep snow. Maybe he had found my Bear Paws on the deck. He was apparently shooting his footage from several feet off to the side of my tracks, leaving my actual path undisturbed. I'm sure the investigators appreciated the courtesy.

"And here we see the big tree where you landed, and the hole where you dropped and slid along the forest floor beneath the snow... and here, the hole where Mark dug you out as the lone survivor of the Falling Skies."

It was unnerving. How did she get this footage even before the investigators arrived? How did I ever dig such a big pit in my weakened and drunken condition... with just a snowshoe? How did I manage to haul him out?

"Any thoughts, now that you've seen the site?" The cameras returned to a live feed from the hospital room.

"Yes. I think—no, I *know*—that the Lord is good. The Lord has love... and power. The power to judge, and the love to save. Our job is to hear... and then to boldly obey. He will do the rest. There is always a way with the Lord."

"I guess after what you've survived, such enthusiastic optimism and faith is to be expected."

"I should think so!" He laughed.

"And what are the doctors saying? What have they found? Broken bones? Ruptured organs?"

"None. Just a very sore hip, receding nips of frostbite, and these bandages. My face took the worst of it."

"You were wearing a thick parka?"

"Yes. I was flying to Chicago to speak at a special Palm Sunday 'Return of the King' conference. The Midwest had just been hit with a big spring snowstorm."

Saundra nodded. "Many flights were canceled or delayed."

"Correct. I was one of the passengers to be rerouted. Oringinally, I was not even booked to be on that flight."

"Amazing."

"A few minutes before the explosion, I felt a deep, dark sense of doom. I actually started to physically shiver, almost violently. When I couldn't shake that icy chill, I stood and retrieved my parka from the overhead compartment above my seat. I'd brought the parka because of the snowstorm."

He took a sip of water.

"As I finished zipping—before I sat down—the plane was ripped apart by the first explosion, near the back of the plane. Immediately, I was in the air. Thankfully, I was now in my parka, plummeting so fast in such thin air that I couldn't really breathe at first. The second explosion, a much larger one, occurred right after I'd been thrown clear."

"Actually," said Saundra, "investigators are speculating that there were numerous small explosive devises strategically positioned throughout the plane. They were all synchronized. Fortunately for you, the device near the tail of your plane detonated a couple seconds prematurely, and that's what saved you."

"Yes, God saved me." There was a little swagger in his voice. Perhaps a bit of humor. "It was a Freak Fall Miracle... from God."

"Who is in a position to argue with that?" She smiled. "And your face? What are the doctors saying about your face?"

"The doctors don't know. They think it will be a long and slow recovery. They are shocked I didn't lose one or both eyes. They say plastic surgery will help... up to a point." He touched two fingers to the gauze. "Yes, I must apologize for my rather unnerving appearance. Thankfully, these bandages will come off tomorrow."

"They will be changing your bandages daily?"

"No. I mean after tomorrow, I will no longer need them."

Saundra straightened.

"I hadn't heard that. I was told your facial injuries were extensive. Not only your skin, but deep tissue injuries, as well as some nerve and circulation damage."

"True. On the other hand, if God has a plan, hang on. It's already a done deal."

"God has healed you already?"

"Not yet. Phase One healing began immediately for all of the bruises and spots of frostbite. And for all of the minor wounds throughout my body. And for the deep tissue injuries. Tonight is the miracle for my face. Tomorrow, I'll be removing these wraps and walking out of here like Lazarus... healed from the grave."

I shook my head at the screen. Bonkers. Brain damaged for sure. Poor Ms. Paige. She awkwardly shifted in her chair, nervously bouncing an involuntary glance off her cell phone, which had somehow drifted into her left hand.

"Healed?"

"Fully healed."

"Normal?"

"Oh, I doubt that," he laughed. "What I mean is, tomorrow I will have no further need for all of this." He waved his arm in a grand gesture, starting with his facial bandages and expanding to his room and the entire hospital.

The bizarre spectacle of this pretty young media personality interviewing an expressionless face wrap—a certifiable religious nut job—was beginning to take its toll. The integrity of everyone involved would soon be on the line. Yet there was no indication of pressure from off camera to call the interview short. Perhaps the director and producer were as spellbound as I was, wondering what might come next. Wondering how much stranger the interview could possibly get.

"Yes," resumed Saundra, her voice wavering only slightly, "God surely is all-powerful. And you were blessed to survive. I would not doubt that in time, you will be healed."

"Amen to that." His head bobbed twice. "Tomorrow."

"So..." she shot a quick glance off camera, then back. "What was it like as you were falling? They say you never blacked out on the way down, only after you hit? I've been told that you say you saw... angels?"

"Yes," he leaned forward, almost reaching to touch her hand, as if about to share a juicy bit of gossip. "And I heard them. They were singing over me all the way down. The angels promised I would live, and that God was setting me apart for a very special assignment."

"And that assignment is...?"

"This, right here and now. And what is yet to come."

"My interview..." she smiled, feigning embarrassment towards one of the profile cameras, "talking to me tonight is your assignment from God?"

This was where the bottom fell out. Too bad the feed was live. Certainly the networks would have preferred a much shorter pause, and a completely different reply.

Saundra nodded, trying to coax a response. Without looking down, she unconsciously pulled the stylus note pen from her phone and tapped it against the phone's dark case.

"Sir?" she wheedled. "You mentioned an assignment from God."

She waited a few more moments for his answer, then abruptly sat backwards when it finally arrived.

"I need to share a warning." He turned from her to the closest camera.

"More will die. Millions."

The pause was now in Saundra's lap. To her credit, she hung in there.

"Millions?" A hint of incredulity colored her response. She mustered an air of professional condescension. "Certainly you have no way that you can...."

"Millions. Soon."

"That's a bit of a shocking speculation, Reverend Jacobs."

"Freak. You must now call me Freak."

"Freak?"

"Yes. It was a Freak Fall Miracle, and I am Freak. God has instructed me to now use this name."

"As you wish... ah... Freak."

"Thank you. And yes, as I said, more disasters are coming. Worse than what we've just seen. Starting within a week."

She shrugged, clearly wondering now how much longer her producer would let this continue. She suddenly seemed almost desperate to have someone pull the plug.

I closed my eyes against the screen. Stood. Sat. Swore at the embarrassing fool.

"Freak," she implored, "it is a potentially dangerous thing to make such a prediction in front of a live viewing audience this way. Our president has declared a state of emergency. People around the world are already terrified, grieving, confused, angry. Cities are in chaos. Fires still rage in several places throughout Europe. Borders have been closed."

"I wish it were not so. I wish I could give some answer other than this." His voice dropped almost to the same whisper I had heard earlier in the day. "I only speak God's truth."

Saundra dabbed a finger to her ear jack, hesitated, then pressed ahead.

"Is this a private theory, or do you have information that might be of use to Homeland Security? Or helpful to the military?"

"There is nothing anyone can do."

"How can you be so sure of your predictions?"

"Scientists, geologists, and even sociologists... they all make predictions. When a prophet of God declares something, it is forewarning. Just as surely as a whistling tea kettle tells you what you'll find when you lift the lid, so I am declaring that judgments are already in motion. Things are coming to a boil even as we speak."

"Freak... you say you are a prophet. A prophet of doom. Would you say you're more like Noah, or more like Jonah?"

He hesitated, clearly weighing his response.

"That, Ms. Paige, may very well be the most difficult question—and perhaps the most critically important question—I've ever been asked. Noah foretold of global destruction, and it came to pass. Jonah warned of total destruction of the wicked... but the people repented... and they were spared."

"And... which is it? Noah... or Jonah?"

He cleared his throat. "I am not sure. God has not yet made it clear to me."

Saundra leaned, perhaps sensing an opening.

"You say you are a prophet, but you don't really know what is coming. Perhaps our viewers need not worry too much about...."

"I have seen the destruction. It is to be. By this time next weekend, the world will have proof that I speak for God. And that Jesus Christ is bringing down the hammer and demanding that the world repent. He is demanding we turn from the pursuit of happiness... to the pursuit of holiness."

"Are you saying God does not want us to be happy?"

"God knows what true happiness is, and God knows better than we about how we can effectively attain it. Most of us do not have a clue. Jesus wants us to know joy, and he knows that most of us are currently on a path that ends in ruin and death. As I said, Jesus is bringing down the hammer on history because he loves us. We need to pay attention to whatever blows may come, and we must respond to these disasters with repentance and a humble pursuit of holiness. Not cursing. Not denial."

"Tell me again... how do you know about these impending disasters?"

"I know, because God has shown them to me. God told me."

"Ah," she sighed with exaggerated relief. "God told you."

"Yes."

"And God told you this... before or after you hit the tree?"

Her question came off as a declaration, as a dismissal of Freak as a crackpot.

During the long moment Freak took to formulate his reply, the lovely Saundra was anything but pretty. I almost felt sorry for Freak. Then again, only hours before, it had been me making the cracks about the arrogant lunatic landing on his head.

"We are almost done here, Ms. Paige. I sense you are a good woman, and you want to do what's right." He drilled straight into her eyes. "I will forgive you for the murderous tone with which you asked that question."

Despite thick makeup, her face turned a stony gray.

"Ms. Paige, I appreciate your professionalism and your humanity in wanting to protect your audience from unwarranted hysteria. I must repeat, however, that millions more will die. You are right, though, that chaos and hysteria are not what is required. What the Lord requires is this: that we act justly, that we live a life of mercy, and that we humble ourselves before our Creator and Judge. The world needs to repent and obey."

"You're quoting the Bible."

"Yes. Micah 6:8. 'He has shown you, O mortal, what is good. And what does the Lord require of you? To act justly and to love mercy and to walk humbly with your God.'"

"Very familiar verses."

"Very neglected verses."

"Surely, as a pastor you know there are times to challenge people, and there are times to comfort them. Right now, the world needs a good shepherd. The story of your incredible survival, your miracle, is a bit of good news in the midst of a global tragedy. The world needs to be reassured that things will be all right. Reverend Jacobs, your miracle survival is the kind of story we need. Right now, the world needs tender words of encouragement and hope, not an incitement to fear and trembling."

"Please, call me Freak. And right now, what the world really needs is an urgent plea and a heavy dose of truth. The ax is laid to the root of the tree."

"How can you quote those sorts of scriptures at a time like this? How about Psalm 23, 'Yea, though I walk through the valley of the shadow of death, I will fear no evil, for thou art with me... Thy rod and thy staff they comfort me....'"

"Now," he interrupted, matching her intensity, then surpassing it, "now of all times... *this* is the Final Hour. This is when words of warning *must* be proclaimed. The world has slept beside still waters. A tidal wave is now coming. Unless the nations humble themselves and repent, utter destruction awaits. With death bearing down upon us all, this is *not* the time for politics, let alone a time for nursery games and lullabies."

"Lullabies?" Saundra snapped. "John 3:16... 'For God so loved the world....' Who are you to sow terror and threats? Over 2,000 people died in airplanes around the world yesterday, and an estimated 2,000 more were killed in fires and explosions on the ground. If God was to speak to the world in such a state, God certainly would not...."

Freak cut her short with a wave of his hand.

"Ms. Paige. My wife buys a certain brand of wonderful, soft, absorbent diapers. We love our babies, and when they are innocent and young, we buy them Pampers.

But as children age, we expect them to do better than to simply roll around and cry whenever they want to be changed. We expect them to grow up. As loving parents, we train and demand they begin to rise to their potential... to live the way humans were designed to live. With all of the freedom and mobility and dignity of being diaper free."

Saundra recrossed her legs.

"The problem today," said Freak, "is that many of us want only to be pampered. We throw tantrums and curse God, rather than accept the training required to raise us to our real potential."

"So," responded Saundra. "What you are saying is that we've got a God who is going to start spanking his children? That God is going to kill millions of people as a way to potty train humanity...."

"I have much more to say," sighed Freak. "But now is not the time."

He lifted his hand. "I will speak again, tomorrow. At a press conference. Bandages off. Fully healed, for all the world to see the power of the Lord. Thank you, Ms. Paige. Thank you, world. May God be with you... and may *you*... decide to believe... and to obey."

THE RECAP
7

Television crews scoured the valley throughout the night, hunting down leads for additional wreckage shots and more local color interviews. One of the network teams caught wind of the lodge where I was staying and set up camp in the lobby. I hunkered down behind the double-bolted doors of my second level sprawling suite, taking advantage of the master bedroom steam shower and room service before indulging in a few deep breaths and reengaging with another bottle of wine and the flat screen theater system in the central fireplace room.

Military experts, aviation engineers, sociologists, historians, politicians, seminary professors... streams of opinions flowed relentlessly through every venue imaginable as humanity attempted to make sense of one of the most shocking days in recent global history.

I channel surfed, watching in fascination as Freak's interview was dissected and analyzed line by line by folks who mined their insights from textbooks, past experiences, Facebook pages, blogs, Twitter tweets, and in some cases, from the facts and actual events of the past two days.

From time to time, a bite from my own press conference was spliced into the mix. It was unnerving to see myself trying to be cute in the swirl and chaos of the other clips of carnage and devastation from around the world. A few of the pundits even bothered to comment on me, or what I said. Saundra herself, in passing, referred to me at one point as a "reliable source." I saluted her with my glass and a grin, then offered an appreciative nod to her lovely face on the 70 inch screen.

Again, it wasn't all about Freak. Stories from the other nine crash sites were in many ways more spectacular. Tales and video footage of heroic rescues from burning buildings and wrecked cars flooded the news, balanced by heart-wrenching clips of sobbing friends and anxious family members waiting for dreaded confirmations. Camera phone photos from bystanders at various sites often left me breathless, even closing my eyes.

The Freak interview, though, kept the whole Falling Skies pot churning at an anxious full boil.

Certain clips were repeating on every channel. Through the mummy wrap of Freak's face issued forth the confident claim, "God spared me the sudden stop at the end. He caught me in His arms."

Then there was Saundra's innocent face, her smile melting into horror at his words: "I need to share a warning. More will die. Millions... soon..... Starting within a week."

Commentators were indignant about Freak's potty training metaphor. Several exploded over the analogy being used in conjunction with a declaration that Jesus Christ would bring down the hammer on those who refused to submit to the Christian religion. One woman suggested that the Jesus of Freak's universe was an abomination. A "perpetrator of child abuse." She for one, would have nothing to do with a religion driven by such barbaric themes.

And then there was Freak's incredible and specific prediction: "Tonight is the miracle for my face. Tomorrow, I'll be removing these wraps and walking out of here like Lazarus... healed from the grave."

One of the national anchors put it best, articulating the angst of millions of us who slept little that night. In the most somber of tones, he met our eyes and asked, "What does this mean?"

"This man now calls himself 'Freak.' The Reverend Bill Jacobs built an entire career and a lucrative empire trafficking in End Times paranoia. He tapped into—and elevated—some of the most obscure passages of Christian scriptures. He exploited the deep repressed anxieties we all suffer as each of us wrestles with our own mortality and the horrific threats of global politics, social upheaval, and war. He has been loved and hated by millions for almost a decade.

"And now, he alone lays claim to the impossible." The anchor paused, glanced down at the editorial in his hands, then lifted his gaze.

"This man fell from an exploding plane... and lived to tell. Not a broken bone in his body. Furthermore, this religious leader, now insisting we call him 'Freak,' claims that God Himself somehow held out His arms and caught him in the branches of a pine tree, then lowered him into a pile of soft snow.

"This man elaborates, insisting he was not alone when he plummeted to the earth, but that actual spirits—living angels—sang over him as he plunged to what should have been certain death. He now claims the Creator of the Universe has saved him and given him an assignment for the End of Days. A message of judgment and death for the world... unless we change our ways.

"What are we to make of this?"

The commentator paused. And then, in the most unprofessional or in the most calculated of moves, he licked his lips.

"Of all the people it could have been... this is the only one to have survived."

He slowly lowered his script to the desk, hands trembling.

"Either this makes no sense at all... or the implications are frightening... almost beyond comprehension."

MONDAY

I awoke on the couch with a stiff neck after a few hours of fretful rest. Ignoring the television, I ordered a healthy breakfast and made a few calls using the room's phone. Everyone had seen me on the news, but nobody had been able to reach me. My cell phone was still on the kitchen counter back at the cabin, and I was in no hurry to wade through a dozen news teams to retrieve it.

My mother promised that she was praying for me, even though she knows I hate it when she says that, and she wanted to know if Bill Jacobs was as tall and good looking in person as he is on television. I reminded her of the bandages and that I'd not yet seen him standing, and she got flustered and put dad on the line.

"Mark," he said, his voice in that satisfied tone I'd not heard in years. It was a tone reserved only for special occasions, like when I'd scored a winning point. "My son, you did good. We're proud of you."

"Thanks, Dad."

"Did you remember to lock up the cabin, or should I drive up there myself to put things in order?"

Hmm.

"You forgot to lock the doors, huh?"

"I kinda had my hands full."

"Of course. I'm not criticizing. I understand. Did you have a woman with you? I didn't see any pictures of any women with you. Would it be safe for me to just drive up and take care of the cabin myself?"

"No women. Suit yourself about the cabin. Thanks again, Dad, as always."

I kept the rest of my calls short. My roommate Brian promised to hold the money we won from bets on the games that were played before the airlines went down. Heather said I looked cute on TV, and she fawned about how much she missed me. I called my English department chair and said they should line up a substitute teacher for me, that the trauma really had me rattled.

I told everyone to pass along my updates, and then I finally put the phone aside and turned back to the news.

Things had changed overnight. More data and better back stories began accumulating, and there was less need to fill the gaps with wild guesses and half-baked opinions. Techno-geeks had slaved through the night to work up compelling graphics and simulations on everything from global disaster site grids to fuselage crash trajectories.

The greatest area of speculation remained Freak, and even there, the sidebars and back stories were beginning to throw new light on the situation.

For one thing, come to find out, Freak was not the first guy to survive something like this. Over a dozen people had survived similar free falls without a parachute, including airman Alan Magee from New Jersey.

During World War II, Magee dropped over four miles from a burning B-17 Flying Fortress. He crashed through a French railroad station glass roof and was ripped apart and busted up almost to the point of death. But he did eventually recover. In fact, Magee lived to travel around talking about his fall for another forty years.

Additionally, contrary to what some people almost learned in their high school physics class, Freak would not have fallen at the rate of 32 feet per second squared. At least not after the first 1,500 feet or so. After the initial acceleration, air resistance against Freak's flapping parka probably would have maxed him out at around 120 miles per hour. Thanks to body drag and wind friction, Freak's terminal velocity from the airplane was roughly the same as if he'd been tossed from the roof of a really tall skyscraper.

Of special interest was another survivor, who, like Freak, didn't break a single bone. A network researcher managed to dig out old photos and the story of Flight Sergeant Nicholas Alkemade, a British war hero who bailed from a burning plane in 1944 at 18,000 feet. The guy didn't have a parachute, but like Freak, he fell through tree branches and landed in snow. He even walked away in better shape than Freak, with only a sprained leg and a Gestapo interrogation, having fallen behind enemy lines rather than onto a primetime news platform.

Both World War II stories came with impressive documentation, leading a surprising number of pundits to the conclusion that surviving an airplane fall without a parachute is not that big of a deal.

Other commentators were less objective.

Unapologetic critics claimed that Bill Jacobs was certifiably unstable and untrustworthy—even dangerous—long before the fall. Numerous failed predictions in recent years put him on the outs with many former allies, including several respected religious groups and a half dozen high-profile academically credentialed leaders. Some of these entities were now coming out of the woodwork, going on the record, and issuing a legion of rather unsavory statements to the press. A couple of radical groups went so far as to claim that Freak was Satan's prophet for the Anti-Christ.

The pastor's surprisingly obese wife, Ellen Jacobs, appeared bug-eyed and distraught on the morning news. A local television station had caught her last night in a frumpy housedress. She refused to make a statement, and she appeared dazed and overwhelmed while shown unloading her kids from an old minivan in the family's dark driveway. She swayed awkwardly, raising her hand against the white glare of a camera light, trying to herd several small children through the front door of their modest home. Her only comment: "Leave us alone."

I turned it off in disgust. The phone rang.

"Mark, it's me. Freak."

I took a deep breath.

"How's the room, Mark? Did I tell you they would hook you up, or what?"

"Yeah, the room is nice. Are you still planning on moving over to here tonight? I've got your keys." I shifted the receiver to my other hand. "But I am thinking that I might be heading back down to Denver this afternoon."

"What's wrong? You can't.... I need you...."

"Of course I can. And I will. I saw your interview with Saundra last night. You really roughed her up at the end when you two started getting personal. Pardon the pun, but when you pulled off the Pampers...."

"Please, " Freak sighed. "I have already taken enough of a beating for that reference."

"Well," I said. "All humor aside, you've got the whole world spooked. If the attacks weren't bad enough by themselves, your interview and your promise that Jesus was going to bring the hammer down was the icing on the cake. The global markets and Wall Street have dropped into a tailspin. And I just saw what the media did to your wife. It's too much. Count me out."

There was another classic Freak pause. I didn't even want to ask if he was still there. I finally started to hang up.

"Mark... listen to me. I know you must be, as you say... spooked."

"Hell-yes."

"Okay, I get that. Give me a few more hours, and that's it. I need you."

"Why me?"

"Because—like it or not—you got drafted. You're now my wingman. At least until I get through this press conference today. I made them bring a TV to my room last night so I could watch the news, and I saw how the whole thing has been playing. I'm in a horrible position right now. And this morning... some of the shows are starting to crucify me. Right?"

"And...?"

"Look, Mark. I'm not saying you have to believe everything I say. But I can feel the tingling heat and the healing of my face happening even as we speak. And you've got to believe what you saw with your own eyes. God saved me for a reason. This miracle wasn't for me... it was for the world."

"Delusions of grandeur," I sighed. "That's what they're calling it. Maybe with some survivor's guilt tossed into the salad to season things up."

"Perhaps. Maybe that's all this is." His voice grew sad, resigned. "You know, Mark... it's pretty hard for a man in a straitjacket to make a case for his own sanity."

"What do you want from me? Am I supposed to confirm that you landed feet first, and not on your head? That's about all you've talked me into at this point."

"Fair enough. Stick with me for a few more hours, and then you can bail before tonight's press conference if you're still not sure. No hard feelings."

"What are you up to?"

"Here's what we need. Get ahold of Saundra for me. Beg her to do another story in my hospital room. She'll listen to you, and she'll have to risk it."

"Why?"

"Because you're my reliable witness. God gave me a reliable witness."

"You know I don't believe in...."

"Exactly. That's why we can all count on you."

"On his head. The poor guy landed on his head...."

"Okay then?"

"What do you want?"

Like a flipped light switch, his tone flashed again with enthusiasm. "I want her here for the drama when we unwrap that long white belt of gauze."

"You're joking?"

"She's gotta be there... in the hospital room... for the unveiling."

"She's gotta be nothing. The only thing for sure she's gotta be is worried that you'll be throwing her more of your curve balls. You embarrassed her last night when...."

"Maybe. But *the big story* is her life of choice. This is who she wants to be. Tell her even if I'm wrong about what I say comes next, the visual documentation of today's miracle will cinch her career in the history books. They'll be showing this footage in journalism classes for years. Last night was incredible. The whole planet saw her amazing live interview."

I held my breath.

"Tell her, I promise... today's story is even bigger."

UNMASKED

She said yes.

It took all of the courage I could muster to call Channel 5, then to wait ten minutes for her to call back, and then finally to argue my case.

Thankfully, Saundra was still in Summit County, over in Frisco doing an interview with a doctor at the hospital. Her manner was a bit brisk and intimidating, so I closed my eyes and imagined I'd just met her in a bar—and she was smiling half way through her third Margarita—even though it was clear from her tone on the phone that she was not the least bit lightheaded. Thankfully, Freak was right. News was her life... but she had her price.

Condition One: No live feed.

Condition Two: Complete editorial and production discretion.

Saundra insisted upon the freedom to work with her director and producer to cut, edit and splice; they could do as much voice-over commentary as they felt necessary, even if that delayed the broadcast uplink by several hours. Apparently, a handful of critics and several of the more competitive local stations were having a field day at Saundra's expense, blasting Channel 5 for the irresponsibility of last night's debacle. She was not about to lose control of an interview and set herself up for such criticism again.

After lunch, as agreed, I passed through security and a growing crowd of out-of-town gawkers. I met two of the hospital's top administrators in the lobby. The rest of the media glared with envy—a few taping and scribbling in notepads—as Saundra and her team were also waved through security to join me in our march back to Freak's central command headquarters upstairs.

Saundra briskly floated down the corridors, clicking her heels as coldly and professionally aloof as she had been on the phone. I tried to connect, making a few jokes that were wasted on everybody except Steve, the rotund mobile cameraman, who seemed to find me hilarious. I invited him over to my lodge townhouse suite for a couple beers after we were done taping. I glanced at Saundra, then magnanimously suggested that he definitely should bring a date.

Our unlikely entourage finally reached the last closed door. We paused for a few minutes outside, catching our breaths and reviewing the plan. And then we entered.

Freak sat expectantly in his baby blue hospital gown. His bed was fully inclined, his hands folded on his lap. Not a single IV. No monitors. A seasoned-looking doctor stood at attention to the left of Freak, reviewing the chart in his hand, barely glancing up as we entered.

Two middle-aged nurses with trays, supplies and instruments flanked and fidgeted from the right. Steve was already recording from his shoulder cam by the time Saundra made her entrance as the last person into the room.

Two administrators produced and explained a variety of documents needing signatures, and a second cameraman quickly began staging a tripod and lights. Freak was polite, articulate, and firm. He acknowledged their many concerns, then waved them off and turned to Saundra.

"Thank you for coming." Freak's voice lathered with appreciation.

"Of course." Saundra glimpsed past Freak to the doctor, then the nurses.

"And Mark, thank you for pulling this all together."

"Just following orders," I smiled. Both cameras were now rolling. I wondered if Saundra would agree with Heather's opinion that I looked cute on film. I decided it didn't matter. I was destined for the cutting room floor either way.

Saundra stepped to the doctor's side of the bed. She shook Freak's hand twice, rather stiffly in my opinion, then took a deep breath and slipped over into her irresistibly beaming self, still holding his hand.

"Your grip is strong this afternoon, Reverend Jacobs." Her clutch lingered, then released in a theatrical farewell to the celebrity's hand. "How are you feeling today?"

"Wonderful, Ms. Paige. Absolutely blessed. But please... do call me Freak."

"Ah, Reverend Jacobs, I would like to honor your request, but I am not in the habit of calling pastors names that sound, so... undignified. Perhaps I could just call you Mr. Jacobs?"

"Thank you, Saundra... may I call you Saundra? But I must insist...."

They went on like that for several minutes, testing each other, wasting film, warming up. At best, only a few seconds of this dueling courtship would end up on the air, but it felt important, and they both seemed to take it very seriously. I realized that when it came to the media and professional personas, I had a lot to learn. I was receiving a crash course from a couple of pros, and it was fascinating. Finally, in some unspoken way, they established an agreement for the tone of the scene to follow, and a consent emerged for the ground rules for the high-stakes game ahead.

"Yes," said Saundra, "I can see that you are no longer on the IV."

"Praise God. The healing continued throughout the night and into the morning. All pain is entirely gone, and I'm ready for the medical staff to remove these bandages. And, for the record, they have been wonderful here. I have nothing but praise for the entire staff here at the Frisco Trauma Center."

"And are you still confident you have been healed?"

"Absolutely. This is not my first healing. In the past, God has used me to heal others. But I, too, was miraculously healed once before." He swung the calf of his right leg out from under the sheet. "Ironically, as a child, I once fell from a tree and suffered a severe compound fracture."

He pointed to a small pink scar.

"I was completely healed in less than 24 hours. As my father prayed over me that night, I felt repeating cycles of intense heat, and then tingling. Just like now with my face. All those years ago, as I rested in my parents' bed, God told me that He was healing me. It was during my first healing episode when I heard God calling me into ministry."

Steve stepped closer and got a tight shot of the scar.

"You were completely healed in one day?" Saundra's voice was gentle, nothing incredulous in her tone so far.

"I never wore a cast. Afterwards, I was climbing trees and playing hide and seek again within three days. And now I've been saved and healed by God once more."

"Doctor?" asked Saundra, drawing the physician from the background into the frame. "In fairness to you and the hospital, I understand you have reservations about this?"

"We've run tests. To the best of our ability, short of removing the bandages, at this point we can find nothing wrong with Reverend Jacobs. To be honest, I find it remarkable. While I do not expect to find his face healed, I'm astonished by his survival from the fall and his amazingly swift recovery. Mr. Jacobs has signed over to us legal permission to talk freely about his injuries and his present condition. He has encouraged us to speak openly, so I must say, I've never seen anything like his case, right from the first hour he was admitted."

"In what way?"

"His pain management. Incredible. The normalization of his blood counts, astounding. Every bone, ligament and joint intact. Hemoglobin, hematocrit... everything essential was fully restored overnight. His reduction in facial swelling and the healing of the bruises on his arms and legs...."

"Thank you, doctor," said Freak. "The Lord has been busy."

"Sir," asked Saundra, clearing her throat, "as a licensed physician, what do you expect to find beneath the bandages?"

"Upon the patient's request, we've only changed his dressings once since he arrived. That is, shortly after his admission, we removed the emergency dressings that had been applied to stem the bleeding, and we replaced them with these."

The doctor passed a hand over Freak's wraps.

"Because the patient has been conscious and fully coherent, and because there has been no compelling medical reason to override his wishes, it's been a day since we've seen his wounds. I'm not at all positive about what we'll find...."

"Again," said Freak, his voice insistent, "I thank you for the exemplary quality of your medical attention throughout my entire visit. But I am now eager for my discharge. I have much to do yet today in preparation for tonight's global press conference. It is time for the removal of this shroud."

"Pastor... Freak," smiled Saundra, "your eagerness to speak to the world is a curious thing. Before we proceed, given that we don't know what to expect...."

"Yes, we do. I've been healed. I've already made this clear."

"Yes," she nodded, "you have. Please indulge me. One more question, please, and then I will step back and let the medical staff begin."

He studied her eyes, then agreed.

"America," she said, "is reeling from recent events. Yet you seem very eager to claim God wants you to prophesy doom, and to predict that more disasters are on the way. It would seem to me that a pastor's job...."

Freak lifted his hand. "I think," he said, "that you had a question for me?"

Saundra shifted. "Are you certain God has called you to be a prophet for the End Times, or is it possible that because of the shock of the explosion and your fall, and all of the trauma you've been through...."

Freak again lifted his hand.

"I am certain," he said, a hint of impatience in his voice. "There is no doubt God has anointed me to speak his truth in this season of shaking. The fact that I am sitting here today as the lone survivor of the Falling Skies Massacre is a proof of my calling by God into this role." He pointed at his face.

"And this will be the confirmation."

Saundra smiled. "There can be no doubt you've been saved from what could have been a horrible death. Many people see you as a sign of hope, an affirmation that someone is always watching over us, even when things go badly."

"The West," said Freak, "has a perverted idea of God. Most people are led to believe that God is either dead, or he is a Santa Claus who listens to our wish lists and does the best he can to love, love... love."

"But," said Saundra, "the Bible does say God *is* love...."

"Yes. But the word *love* has often been reduced in the West to needlepoint. The Bible also says God is holy. And full of wrath. And not to be mocked. And yet quick to forgive. God is not a bumper sticker slogan, Ms. Paige. He is almighty. He is complex. He is sovereign over history. And he gets to call the shots."

"And what do you say to the other pastors and the millions of people of faith who believe some of those primitive understandings of God and the Bible have now been corrected through time by...."

"Saundra. Let us debate this another time. I will close now with one final thought."

He turned from her and leaned toward the camera held by Steve.

"I believe it was the Protestant Reformer Martin Luther who gave us a litmus test of sorts for determining the authenticity of a religious leader. Luther's question was, quite simply:

Does the pastor know of death and the Devil?
Or is it all sweetness and light?"

Freak turned to the doctor.

"Let us get on with this. Thank you for your patience."

The doctor shrugged at Saundra, who immediately busied herself muttering final instructions to the rest of her team. The tripod moved closer. Steve slipped around to the other side of the bed. A light was adjusted.

Freak closed his eyes.

He pulled two deep breaths, sufficient to draw the room into his silence. Slowly, he lifted his right hand high over his head, toward the ceiling and beyond.

Then he softy slid into a low, indecipherable prayer.

In the midst of that quivering—those quiet little gestures—a sense of something sacred and monumental entered the room. I think we all felt it. Turning from Freak, I observed Steve recording, but he appeared to be holding his breath, his head oddly tipped, staring around the camera, not through it.

Freak finished, lowered his hand, and then opened his wet and expectant eyes. Both cameras and everyone in the room zoomed their focus tight to his face.

Saundra whispered to the doctor that she would not distract him or the nurses by trying to talk during the procedure. She would forfeit any attempt at a running commentary, and instead, she would generate a voice-over narration later, as needed. She absently pulled the stylus from the bottom of her cell phone and opened her note app, nodding to the doctor and each of the nurses, who hesitantly nodded back.

Freak asked them to begin.

The medical team positioned their tray and instruments, then pulled forward a stainless steel hazardous waste receptacle. Slowly, precisely, they began to unwrap. Saundra leaned forward as spellbound as the rest of us, swaying an inch or two closer, then back, each time the doctor's arm completed an orbit around his head.

As the last of the wrappings were removed, all that remained were three large sterile bandage pads. They were darkly stained, overlapped and crusted together. They covered the entire left side of Freak's face, from his stubbled square jaw up past his thick left eyebrow and into his greasy black hair.

The doctor dabbed two of his gloved fingers into a dish of gel, then began to gently pry and lift and withdraw the mask.

Later, the attending physician was willing to go on record with Saundra that as far as he knew, such a rapid open wound recovery of this magnitude was virtually without published precedent... medically impossible. As far as he was concerned, this actually did qualify as a miraculous healing of some sort.

The bad news: the cameras caught it all... and Freak's face was hideous.

Several of us gasped.

Even the nurses swayed slightly as they received from the doctor the last of the mask. Again, later, after all of the gel and ointments and crusted blood and dried puss was wiped away, his face was not as horrific as it first seemed. Still, the troughs and ridges of raw facial scar tissue that flamed in grotesque purples, reds and pinks would for months force those with weak stomachs to look away.

Freak read the reactions around the room. He closed his eyes, then waited until they were finished cleaning his face. His breathing became fast and shallow, and much too loud for the now deathly quiet room.

The doctor started to say something, then let it go.

The sloshing of the water and sponges in the basin grew to an obscenely loud focused distraction. The nurses squeezed the last of the wash and rinse from their final sponge. They pulled off their gloves, drew back, then waited with the rest of us, awkwardly suspended somewhere between professional fascination and pedestrian revulsion.

Eventually, Freak pointed to the hand mirror waiting atop a table nearby.

He lifted the mirror and looked, holding it by the base at arm's length. He flipped it to the magnifying side, then drew it very close. He took one final long gaze, squeezed his eyes, then thrust the mirror out blindly to whoever might remove it from his hand.

He sank slowly back into his pillow, softly muttering unintelligible prayers... or curses.

Perhaps both.

"Saundra, can I buy you a drink?"

She searched my eyes for the first time since we'd met.

"Uh, no. Thanks." She glanced at her tightly circled crew, then down the hospital corridor in both directions, then back to Freak's closed door. "What happened in there?"

She was shaking, ever so slightly. Had I not been at her elbow, I might not have caught her tremors.

"Who knows?" I said, softly. "Maybe we should talk this through...."

She looked up, then turned to Steve. "Did you get it all?"

"Everything. But I'm not sure what we're going to do with it."

She turned back to me. "Thanks for the offer, Mark. You're his friend, right?"

I lifted my shoulders in an noncommittal shrug.

"Yes." She shook her head no. "Let's talk. But not right now. We've got to get this back to the truck. We've got to put something together for tonight's news. Thank God I've got a crack team in the van...."

"Listen," I said. "Bring your guys by my place at the Elkhead Lodge later tonight. We can all watch the finished product together live from there. The suite is swank, and I've got plenty of room."

I turned away from Saundra to the others. "They have probably got you staying at some cut-rate motel... probably some roadside dump with a tarped-over pool, right?"

"Right," said Steve. "It's a real dive. The breakfast is awful, and they've got us all doubled up. And the rooms are way too small. But it's the only thing they could find on such short notice."

"It's settled then. Come up when you can. I've got four bedrooms, a jacuzzi, and two steam showers. I'll leave a light on."

"Crap," she sighed, looking past me again to Steve. "What are we going to do with this? I'm not sure this is what the world needs right now. I'm at a loss...."

"Hold on," I interrupted. "What's the problem here?"

I started to reach for her shoulder, but I lost my nerve and swung wide to knuckle bump Steve's big arm instead. "Folks, you've got another High-5-at-Five exclusive. Freak cancelled his big global press conference, so now you've got today's only show in town. He's spending another night hidden in hospital seclusion by his own request... and the whole planet is waiting for what you alone can show and tell."

I turned back to Saundra. "You guys go to the van and work your magic. Let your producer earn his big bucks. This is the most compelling story in the world tonight, and it's all yours. Relax. Have some fun. Enjoy the good life. Come by the lodge when you can, and I'll pop some cold champagne when I hear you at the door."

A smile flickered across her lips. Her first smile just for me.

"Sure," she said. "But it'll probably be pretty late."

10
CHAMPAGNE

Saundra and Steve didn't arrive until long after Freak's hospital story created another five o'clock sensation.

Apparently, several big shots at the local and network levels phoned in their enthusiastic accolades within minutes of the airing, and the celebrations had begun early. After the second round, a few members of the crew headed from the bar in Frisco back down to their homes in Denver.

By the fourth round, the roadside motel started looking like the best option for the rest.

In the end, only Steve and Saundra decided to risk a weaving drive back up to Breckenridge to spend the night with me.

I heard Steve in the hall before he knocked. Saundra lugged a huge rolling pullman, and Steve wobbled sideways beneath the burden of two black gear bags and an oversized duffle.

"Strictly business," she laughed. A rich drink or two still wafted from her breath. "But the boss says I don't have to clock back in until Freak makes his next move. Maybe tomorrow afternoon? Whatcha think?"

"We'll see," I smiled, bobbing my head and helping her through the door. "Maybe we can pick him up and walk him to lunch tomorrow for some man-on-the-street reactions to our new zombie friend's face."

I reached for the handle of her luggage.

"Then again," I said, "maybe they'll put the Freak on a suicide watch. After what you filmed, if I was him, I wouldn't crawl out from my hole for another three days. If ever."

Saundra winced. Then glared.

"Just kidding," I apologized. "Freak will bounce right back. He's already proven himself to be an invincible hero." Her eyes softened, slightly. "And let's not forget," I added, "Freak says he's got angels at his side."

Saundra hesitated, nodded. Then laughed.

Thankfully, she tittered past me so quickly I was able to shake it off and regroup with a quick gulp behind her back. I'd not imagined she'd be so sympathetic towards the man who'd unnerved her so badly live on the air.

I wheeled her luggage into the suite, then helped Steve navigate his bulk over to the couch. He unceremoniously flopped longwise, then promptly fell to snores.

The muted central living room flat screen still glowed, flickering with news from around the world, including frequent clips from the Saundra and Freak Show. She paused, mildly interested, whenever her face appeared on the screen; she seemed awkwardly indifferent whenever Freak's raw-scarred visage flashed briefly near each segment's end.

Fortunately, by using two cameras, they'd been able to splice together a sequence cutting to Freak's good side and keeping the worst of his face somewhat obscured while filming the last of his dressings being removed.

At one point, I briefly turned the volume much louder. A radical group with Mid-Eastern ties was claiming credit for the attacks. According to their BBC translator, they were declaring their foaming-at-the mouth resolve to utterly finish what they'd begun. They would soon again make the world safe for demagoguery.

Saundra and I filled another half hour of conversation with a bottle of champagne. Our topics rambled and lurched, with probably nothing she'd recall the next day.

I appreciated the time with her immensely, though, as it gave me a chance to get over some of the intimidation I felt while being so close and alone with her. I'd admired her on television for over a year, and she was the first established Hollywood type I'd ever sat with on a couch.

My others had all been novices and wanna-be's.

Even on the verge of passing out, she recorded a list of tomorrow to-dos on her cell phone note pad, and she remained more articulate than several of my previous girlfriends could have faked at the top of their games.

Her voice exhibited a range and bouncing feminine beauty as mesmerizing as the rest of her package.

Saundra had studied journalism in Louisiana, where an internship evolved into a paid spot on the air.

Within a year, she leveraged her way up to the much more prestigious Denver market. And now this story of a lifetime had fallen into her lap, almost as it had in mine.

During another loop of the news, she let slip that her station was assigning her and Steve to stick with me in order to stay as close to the breaking news as possible. The Freak Fall Miracle story was theirs to ride... hopefully all the way to an Emmy.

I poured a couple more glasses of champagne, got an eyeful whenever she looked away, and then finally showed her upstairs to her master suite in the loft. Helping her up the stairs, she missed a step near the top, and I managed to get an arm under her. She was heavier than I expected. Apparently she carried some muscle under all those curves. My investigations were cut short when we reached the cozy fireplace lounge at the top landing. The door to her suite was open, and she gasped at the extravagance of it all. Together we navigated the loft's furniture as I led her into the room. She squirted from my arm when I reached for the light, then danced beyond my reach.

"The jacuzzi is over there," I pointed. "I'll bet you're really feeling tense and sticky after such a big day?"

She laughed.

In a final pirouette, she threw herself onto the king bed in giggles.

She begged me to bring up her luggage. I emphatically promised I would. She thanked me repeatedly, in a lovely but sad diminuendo, then slid into oblivion atop the sumptuous comforter before I could conjure a closing line.

I retrieved her suitcase, took a final inventory of the bed, then killed her light.

11 TUESDAY

I refilled Saundra's tall champagne flute from the mimosa carafe, smiling and agreeing about the magnificence of our balcony view. I reheated my coffee from the service cart and returned to the couch.

It was hard to guess if she'd calculated the effect her adorably smudged makeup would have upon my heart rate. Perhaps she'd planned it. Then again, maybe she'd simply rushed from the loft when I'd opened the door for the breakfast service. Perhaps she'd heard the fumbling locks and feared I was slipping out for adventures with Freak, leaving her—and her Emmy—behind.

"So," I asked, stirring my cup. "How did you manage to find my cabin and to beat the feds to the crime scene?"

"Lucky for me, your cabin isn't technically a crime scene." She took a half-hearted sip from the crystal glass.

She carefully returned her glass to the low table to her left. "We might have gotten into trouble if a crime had actually been committed at your property. Thankfully, I guess, the work of the terrorist was all in the air."

"You didn't know that when you started filming." I shook my finger. "Actually, trespassing *does* make it a crime scene. Not to mention a possible civil lawsuit from me for invasion of privacy by broadcasting footage of my back deck—including potentially incriminating empty beer bottles—without my permission."

"Oh, yeah," she said. "Your sexy beer labels. What a colorful touch they made for an otherwise boring story." She flashed an ironic, flirtatious smile. "You have no idea what a gift you are to my career. I can't wait to see what you come up with for me today." She pretended to shuffle and scan the hotel literature on the coffee table. "Perhaps you have some exotic beach brochures around here that might make for an interesting tight shot?"

"Don't change the subject," I smiled back.

With her hair unbrushed, I couldn't decide whether she was a brunette with dramatic highlights, or a blonde with trendy black lowlights. Either way, it worked.

"By the way" I added. "Thanks for not zooming in too closely on those bottles. My mother watches the news. She would have blushed."

Saundra smiled. "Any decent lady would have blushed. I know I did." She added enough Southern inflection to almost make *me* blush.

Saundra's phone pinged with another message. She ignored the intruder and lifted her plate of half-finished breakfast instead.

"Back to your scoop." I reached into the linen-lined basket and retrieved a pastry from the cart. "How'd you get all of your live footage from the hospital? You must have been there before the story even broke."

Saundra fiddled with her fork as her phone pinged yet again. She nibbled a bite of omelet, then slid everything onto the table next to her unfinished juice.

"Well, we were done with our festival story up in Breckenridge. We had just left Breck and were almost down to Frisco when the explosions occurred. National news from all of the attacks started flooding in through the Denver stations...." She glanced at her napkin, then shuttled it from her lap to the discarded plate. "We were stunned. The thought of thousands of people in the air... hundreds falling right here in the valley near where we were...."

"Did you get any of it on film?"

"No, of course not. Nobody did. Who could have known? At that point, Flight 696 was just another random spot in the sky."

"Not to me. As you know from my press conference... I was looking straight at it when it blew."

After a moment, Saundra resumed.

"At this point, your description is still our best anchor for the front end of this story. Unless someone else steps forward, you're the only one who was watching when it happened. By the time the sounds of the explosions reached the ski slopes... when folks started looking up...."

"That," I said, "is why the investigators were all so relentless in wringing me dry at the hospital."

"Yes. Denver radar showed the WestAir Express Flight flying exactly according to its flight plan until the very moment they dropped from the grid. No warning transmissions, no unusual conversations. Nothing."

"The black box?"

"Not yet. They've located the signal. Mountain Rescue is doing their best to retrieve it. Maybe sometime tomorrow." Her phone pinged again, a different tone this time. "Sorry," she said. "This is one I have to take."

She lifted her phone, found the screen, then quickly scanned through several messages. In one fluid motion, she removed her stylus and jotted a quick note on a fresh digital page.

Outside, the alpine slopes were stirring to life. A few fluffy butt-dragging beginners were already gouging SOS's on the bunny hill. A speeding trio of fluorescent ski bombers raced neck-and-neck, and a pair of boarders floated wide, tacking to the moguls at the edge of the run.

"Okay," she sighed. "Sorry." She put her phone on vibrate and placed it beside her plate and glass. "I hate that thing, but what can I say?" The elegant black and silver stylus lingered in her right hand, gracefully playing baton games over and around her shapely digits.

"Anything urgent from the boss?" I asked.

"More of the same." Her stylus grew still. "Everybody wants information. The top stories from around the world are bleak. More violence. More fear. More dangerous threats from every side. Prayer vigils at the crash sites. And two new terrorist clips have now gone viral."

"Saundra, you're really bringing me down."

"That's my job. And it's been said I do it well."

"On a lighter note," I grinned, "next weekend, we're supposed to get another four inches of powder up here."

"And?"

"Well, maybe, if you're still around, I could show you a few of my favorite runs."

"I'm a pro on the news. On the slopes... not so much."

"Perfect. Then powder is exactly what you need."

She hesitated. "A soft landing might help. Let's give it a few days, then see where we're at."

She smiled.

I needed a moment to regain my thoughts.

"Saundra, you were saying that after you'd finished filming the festival in Breckenridge...."

"Sure. So there we were, topping off our gas tank next to the hospital in Frisco. I was trying to interview a few customers at the pumps, hoping for some local color on the crash story. All of a sudden, I heard a blaring horn. Then you came blasting off I-70. I spotted you running stoplights, so I knew something was big. I shouted for my team to catch what they could as you flew by. Instead, they filmed you slamming brakes and skidding into the hospital parking lot only a stone's throw from our van."

"Lucky you." I almost patted her knee. "And then you sent Steve over to film me unloading the Freak, right?"

"Of course. Neither you nor the victim were dressed for skiing, so I didn't believe for a minute his face was messed up from hitting a tree on the slopes. You were staggering, apparently drunk, and hardly making any sense. There was quite a lot of blood. I heard you mumbling from beside your SUV about the Gore Range. The medic wanted to know where it happened, and you said something about up above Silverthorne. So as soon as the hospital locked us out, I headed over to Silverthorne with the best half of my team. Those we left behind watched for news at the hospital door."

"There are a lot of cabins around Silverthorne."

"Right. But you were falling-down drunk, remember? So I knew you were a serious drinker. We headed straight for the first bar off the highway."

"Brilliant."

"On the drive over, I had my cameraman freeze a clean frame of your face—pre-vomit and *sans* dribbles— and then we printed out a dozen mug shots there in our broadcast truck before we even arrived."

"Absolutely brilliant."

"I walked into the bar and promised a cash reward for my first solid lead. I needed to know who you were, and where you lived. I would pay $200 for anything of use."

"Saundra," I grinned. "You could have saved yourself a lot of time and money. You should have just followed me into the hospital. You could have said you were my girlfriend. They would have taken you to my room, and I would have told you anything you wanted to hear."

"Funny." She shook her head. "I told folks to start with all the bars and liquor stores, because the guy in the photo was a real boozer." She winked. "People quickly fanned out in all directions, armed with copies of your photo in one hand, and copies of my business card in the other. Within 30 minutes, I got a cell phone call from one of my barroom detectives. A college kid hit pay dirt at a liquor store on the edge of town."

"Last Stop Liquors."

"How did you guess?"

"And did you pay?"

"Huh?"

"The college kid. Did he get his two hundred bucks?"

"Well...."

"You didn't have it on you, right? And you gave him an I.O.U.?"

"Channel 5 will mail him a check next week."

I shook my head.

"The clerk off Highway 9 recognized your photo immediately. She was able to tell us your name was Mark Hanson, and she said you mentioned the other day you were heading up for some snowshoeing off Bootlegger Lake."

Hmm. Interesting. She must have checked my credit card receipt. Fair enough. A few of her bottles were probably still sunning on my deck table. Call it even.

"And, Saundra, did you pay her?"

"Well...."

"Never mind."

"You'll be happy to know," she said, "that we *did* pay the guy who drove us to your cabin in his jeep. Some old hippie heard us talking, and he assured us that our Channel 5 truck would never make the climb. He said our uplink dish would snag on low branches, and our city tires would spin us into the ditch. We gave him a fifty dollar bill, and he knew right where to go."

"Probably to the Big Dillon Muddy Pub."

"Huh?"

"Did he have a white beard... ponytail down to here?"
She nodded. "Congratulations, Saundra. You met the once

world-renowned Eddy McGriff. Played a mean guitar and chased a lot of skirts, back in the day. I'm sure your pretty eyes and fifty bucks stirred some good memories... and left a fine taste in his mouth."

"Anyway, he knew the terrain. There weren't a whole lot of fresh tire tracks up there. And only one cabin on Rock Creek Road had an empty driveway with fresh snowshoe tracks all over the place."

"Good work, Watson. And then," I grinned, "when nobody answered the front door, you took it upon yourself as a Good Samaritan to walk around to my back deck for a wellness check. Making sure nobody else was hurt, right?"

"Sorry about the trespassing." She touched the blunt end of her stylus to her lips. Then batted her lashes. "Do you plan to sue?"

"No," I winked, "but you owe me... big time."

The sound of cranking faucets drifted from the bathroom. The hissing water stopped, and Steve made the noises of exiting the shower. A few minutes later he joined us, hair still dripping, grabbing his plate and juice from the cart on his way to the opposite wing of the sectional.

"These robes are amazing," he said, tugging the collar of his plush white terry. "Can I keep this?"

"Sure," I said. "It's on me. It's all on me."

Saundra shook her head.

"What," I objected, "you don't believe I can afford this?"

"I know better," she smiled. "We've got a team of local and network researchers exploring every aspect of this story. Reverend Jacobs is on the verge of personal bankruptcy. And you share a modest little rental with Brian VanDoorn in the cheapest part of town. Even your red gas-hog... the car's title is actually registered in your father's name."

"Please. Don't call her a car. My beastie is an SUV. Insurance is cheaper on my dad's policy. And, for the record, I paid for all of the modifications and accessories myself, right down to the dashboard hula dancer."

"Same with the cabin." She wagged her lovely head. "It's not in your name. Mr. Hanson, you are *definitely* not paying for this executive suite. And you certainly are not buying Steve a robe. You're just a school teacher."

I clutched my heart. "*Just* a school teacher! My lady, I am a purveyor of the most sublime and exquisite literature of all human history. You do me harm... 'tis a mortal wound."

"Okay. So you babysit a high school World Lit class. Don't be such a goof."

"Come on, I have assets."

"Assets? Such as?"

"Well, I've got a new set of Callaway irons. Paid off in full, mind you. I've got two bikes, a Shimano Ultegra road bike for touring, and a Devinci Spartan for off-roading. Still paying on that one, though."

"Keep going, Mark."

"Those Bear Paw snowshoes Steve borrowed... not expensive, but classics. Very hard to find. On Craigslist, I could break even on them in a week. And the sunglasses I wore to watch Freak fall: Oakleys. Top of the line."

"My, you're quite the outdoorsman. What's next? Are you going to give me the rundown on your vast collection of all-weather jock straps? In designer colors, I assume?"

"Dang. You people *are* good! But in truth, it's not so much a collection as an accumulation."

She shook her head. "This has all been very educational. Yes, Professor Hanson certainly is one heck of a teacher. I'm guessing you're fourth generation Ivy League, with trust funds from here to London."

"Ouch. No trust funds. I'm a self-made man. They didn't tell you about my scholarships, did they?"

"Men," she sighed. "They gave you few thousand bucks a year to play ball. Or so your mother says on her Facebook page."

"Yes. But also academic. Did you read how I pulled a double-major, philosophy and literature... *magna cum laude*?"

"My dearest, thou dost protest... too *laude*. Yes, relax. The researchers assured me that you're smart. Very bright. 60 watts at least. On a sunny day, maybe 75 watts... if you're standing by a window."

She turned her grin towards Steve. "How's the steam shower? Did you save any hot water for me?"

"Divine," he sighed, saluting me with his fork. "Thanks for the treat, Mark. I haven't seen so much hot water since the day I called in sick for the Girl Scout Cookie story."

She turned back to me. "Seriously, Mark. Who *is* paying for all of this?"

"Taxpayers?" I shrugged. "I'm really not sure. As I was leaving the hospital, one of the administrators handed me a set of keys and a page from his clipboard. He pointed at the map and instructions, and then he assured me that all the arrangements were in place. He said the suite was mine through the end of the month. Room service. Pantry and bar. The works."

"What about Freak?" asked Steve, reaching for the Mimosa. "He might be broke, but maybe his company or the religious network that runs his shows is paying. I heard his plan was to come up here and stay with you for a few days. He must have known someone else would be picking up the tab."

"Wow," I whistled. "You guys really... really *are* good. How do you come up with that kind of inside information? I could have sworn Freak only shared those plans with me... and only while we were alone. Well, almost alone."

Steve smirked. "Okay if I just finish this?" The carafe was already pressed to his lips.

"Sure," I said, "but it's going to cost you an honest answer. What do you two think of my new friend? As the only two journalists who've actually met the guy since his fall, you've gotta have some kind of opinion. Is this self-declared 'Man of God' the real deal... or is it just his bump on the head that keeps speaking?"

Steve lowered the empty jar.

"Jacobs," he said, wiping his mouth, "he isn't the only religious nut-job in the world. There must be dozens of other fanatics out there right now thinking they've got a hotline to God. Pitching various End of Days scenarios...."

"Granted," I interrupted, "but how many of them have escaped from an exploding airplane in the past week?"

"A minor point." Steve return the carafe to the cart.

"Unlike any other kooks," I said, "Freak has everyone's attention, from the President on down. After what just happened in the skies, people are running scared. Desperate for answers. Listening to Freak. Wondering if this really is the countdown to the end of the world."

Saundra cleared her throat. "I read about a church in Texas sending members into the streets with religious tracts printed to look like airport boarding passes. They're calling them 'Rapture Tickets,' to get past hell and fly straight to heaven when the big day comes."

"Rapture tickets?" I scratched my chin. "So I guess if you pray the lines they printed on the back side, then the next time a plane goes down... you'll go up instead?"

Steve grinned. "Tom Jackson reported on folks saying Jesus is returning any day. The Tribulation has begun."

"Sure," I said. "Anything to fill the Sunday pews."

"He said folks believe a nasty leader will soon be taking over and make us all wear sixes. Then he'll take all our guns and call it world peace. They call him... *The Beast*."

"The Beast," I sighed. "I think I've already met *The Beast*. He lives in South Denver. He told me to leave his daughter alone, and to never knock on his door again."

"Oh," chuckled Steve. "Well, if the Antichrist is from Colorado, then I guess we can ignore the speculation it might be Freak. The Freak is from California."

I laughed. "Aren't they all?"

Saundra flipped her phone and slid the stylus into the bottom slot. She stood and brushed off any invisible crumbs, then looked to the loft.

"I'm going to take a quick shower and put on a fresh outfit. Steve, when I return, you need to be dressed and ready to roll. We've got another big day, and who knows what this afternoon might bring."

She turned to me. "Give it some thought, Mark. It'd be great to have you on our team. Let me know if you can come up with something for us all to do later today. Something worthy of the news."

I smiled, then watched her ascend and disappear through her bedroom door.

12
THE ORANGE
PARKA PLAN

I sensed it was Freak before the second ring.

"It's me," he sighed, his voice raspy, unsure. "Sorry to call so early."

"Good morning," I said, checking my watch. It was almost noon. "How'd you sleep?"

"Not so good. It's been a really hard couple of days and...."

I strained to listen. Saundra's shower was running upstairs, and his voice tapered off until I wasn't sure if he was mumbling or just breathing that hard.

"You'll have to speak up," I said, kindly. "Bill... how can I help you? What do you need?"

"Freak.... it's still Freak."

"Okay." I closed my eyes and tried to picture what I could remember of the unscarred side of his face, to address him there. "I'm really sorry about how things turned out yesterday with the bandages. Are you feeling any kind of pain?"

"Of course I am. But not in my face. Nothing so shallow and simple as that." I glanced in Steve's direction. He'd stopped midbite on a piece of buttered toast. His ear was cocked, and he held his breath to catch whatever he could from the call.

"My face," he sighed at last. "It *was* healed. You know that, right?"

I swallowed hard.

"Look," I coaxed. "I don't know where this is going, but I'm here for you. I want to help. Can I come over to the hospital and get you?"

The softness in my voice, and the wave of genuine sincerity that I suddenly felt, caught me off guard. Maybe it was because I had an open calendar for a few days, and because I was holding a set of keys to one of the most impressive mountain rental properties in the state. Maybe it was knowing that the lovely Miss Paige was upstairs, naked, washing her hair in my shower. I felt... I don't know, territorial or something. For a moment, possessive. Protective.

"It'll be okay," I promised. "Why don't you let me come and get you. I'll bring you back here, and I'll try to help you sort things out."

"Thanks," came the sigh from the other end. "I knew I could count on you."

"How soon can you be ready? I could be there in twenty minutes."

"Make it an hour. I need to wrap up some paperwork with the hospital."

"Deal. See you in an hour."

Steve scarfed the last corner of his toast. Still chewing, he quickly rose and made for his duffle across the room.

"No way," I insisted. "He's already freaking out. The last thing he's going to want to see when he leaves his room is you with another camera jabbing at his face."

"Think about it, Mark. Use your head." Saundra glanced to Steve for support. "There's probably 20 cameras at the hospital locked and loaded already. Probably another 50 reporters already there, just waiting in the parking lot for him to make his next move. Plus, I heard that some protestors or something have started to gather, hoping to somehow connect their crazy agenda to Freak's miracle. There's no way Freak is going to leave the hospital without somebody getting another story."

"She's right," urged Steve. "He's a sitting duck. At least with us, it won't be strangers."

I shook my head. "Uh-uh. He's not ready. You should have heard his voice. I'm telling you, he's a total basket case. If you're right about all the media folks being on stakeout, I'd better find his number and call him back to make a new plan. We could try to get him out tonight, after dark...."

"No. Wait." She sounded desperate. "I've got an idea. Do either of you have a red coat? Or orange? Anything really bright, with a big hood?"

"Sure," I said. "Stuffed under the front seat of my rig. I leave a flashlight, matches, and an emergency parka stashed there all winter. In Colorado, especially in the mountains, you never know."

"Great!" She glanced at the note screen app on her phone, then pointed her stylus at Steve. "You've still got that gaudy Sherpa hat you bought a few days ago at the festival, right?"

"Gaudy?" He grinned.

"No, not the gaudy one," she winked. "I mean the stylish one. The one with the pink elephant earflaps and all of those dangling rainbow tassels."

"It's in my bag."

"Perfect." She drew us in. "Now, I know this is going to sound like an old trick from a low-budget sitcom, but here's what we need to do...."

I don't know what we were thinking.

Yes, I do.

Steve and I were both thinking the same thing: damn, that girl looks good when she gets excited and starts batting her brown eyes. Who could ever say no to *that*?

As planned, we brushed past the media teams stalking around the lodge. When they tried to engage us, we remained tight-lipped, even rude. They cleverly deduced we were up to something important, then obligingly followed us down to the Frisco Trauma Center as if on a leash. During the drive, Steve fetched my neon orange parka from beneath the seat. He donned it with his outrageous hat, and then he really started getting into the charade, making clown faces and bragging about his Lord and Taylor charge account. I pronounced him "King Fool" for the day, and that just juiced him all the more.

The parking lot security guy waved us through, and I settled my SUV in as near as I could get to the Emergency Entrance. Behind us, the trailing pack of live remote vans and media vehicles was diverted to their designated spaces much further out in the frozen slush, beyond the white carnival tent still serving as a makeshift studio and production center for all of the out-of-town teams.

As we unloaded, Steve made a show of himself in his wacky bright outfit, fussing around beside my SUV, waiting for the media crews to stream out from the hospital lobby or to wander in from the hinterlands. He was actually pretty good, pretending over and over to instruct me and Saundra about where we should stand and how we should walk, as if our march to the hospital door was destined to become the most important story ever told.

Once the mob had assembled and grown riotous with questions, Steve hoisted his camera. With his flaps down, it was indeed difficult to see a face. Besides, everyone was—and if necessary would be—aiming their cameras and questions at Saundra and me.

To set the hook, we faked some nonsense about Freak giving us another breaking news exclusive interview in his room upstairs. Then, en masse, we moved the enlisted troops across the lot to the hospital's main entrance, past security, and into the fortified front lobby.

A couple of protestors or fans jeered or cheered as we passed, pumping placards and waving spray-painted sheets demanding Freak's head... or perhaps just a lock of his hair.

Again, as prearranged, security let the three of us through the final checkpoint. Then they held up their arms and restricted the rest. We disappeared down a long hall into the bowels of the building. Steve peddled backwards, recording shoulder-height images of our grins framed by the lobby hordes, who were forced to settle for useless shots of our receding backs.

We turned at the end of the corridor and disappeared several steps down the next hall.

One of the same hospital administrators who had coached me the other day for my press conference stood waiting for us at an open door.

"Is this still the plan, then?" he asked. "Are you sure about this?"

"Yes," I replied. "Unless you can show cause why Reverend Jacobs needs to stay."

"I'd like him to give it another couple more days, but it's his call. It's a patient's right to leave AMA... against medical advice." He turned to Saundra and Steve. "Is everything going okay so far on your end?"

"So far, so good," panted Steve, a bit dizzy from the backwards rush. "Here, take my camera." He shoved it in my direction. It felt lighter than I expected. "Let's hurry," he added, starting to remove the parka and hat as he walked.

We picked up the pace, looping back on another hallway as our guide escorted us towards the Emergency Room. Just outside the ER, Freak stood waiting, watching us approach, his bad side conspicuously turned against the wall.

"Here," said Steve, arriving first. "Put this on."

I drifted to Freak's good side, studying mostly his feet and hands as he took the hat from Steve and fitted it onto his head. He twisted it slightly, until the left flap nearly hid from view his entire left face. He squinted at me and shrugged.

"How do I look?"

"Good." I reached to shake his hand. "Not quite a GQ cover shot, but close."

His grip grew stronger when I finally met his eyes.

"I like it," piped Saundra. "It suits you well. Very subtle. And the lime green tassels really do something for your eyes." She took his hand from mine, pumping his arm like an old friend.

"Yup," said Steve. "That hat has got your name written all over it. It's yours. I'll get another one next year."

Freak smiled. "Thanks. It's Steve, right?" He shook Steve's meaty hand, then turned back to Saundra.

"Ms. Paige, I want to thank you for all that you've done."

"Are you kidding," she smiled. "I'm all mercenary."

"No. You've been kind to me. I tried to use you, and you returned the favor with an honest and fair report. You could have killed me with that second exclusive, and you didn't."

"Let's talk more later," she beamed. "We'll see if you still like me after my third report. I'm not done with you just yet."

"We gotta move," said Steve, gently thrusting the parka between them. "This whole smoke and mirrors escape hinges on speed and the element of surprise."

"Okay then," said Freak, slipping a hand into the coat's dangling sleeve. "Let's do this."

Like an engineer with a beloved design and a well-oiled machine, we had conceived our scheme and were executing the plan with measured precision.

Freak lifted the camera and nestled it against the garish sherpa flap draped over his left cheek. In the glowing orange parka, camera in place, he would pass for Steve, albeit a bit too tall and lean. Steve himself sidled into a back room, off the grid for the next hour or two. Then Saundra would call him forth via her cell phone to fetch him back to the lodge.

Or so we dared to believe.

AMBUSHED

On cue, we charged from the side hallway into the ER. Saundra staggered, faking sobs into a tissue, me draping an arm of reassurance over her shoulder, trying desperately to somehow console her.

Clearly, for all to see, something horrible had happened during Saundra's time interviewing the fallen prophet. Freak played the character role of Steve, the familiar Channel 5 cameraman in orange. He shielded his face with the camera and hat flaps, pretending to record the drama of our traumatic retreat.

Staff and a couple patients appeared surprised and confused, but nobody attempted to detain us as we briskly sniffled our way across the ER and out through the sliding glass doors. We reached my waiting SUV, cleanly, exactly as planned.

That's where our ill-conceived construction zone parka plan came undone.

"Over there!" shouted a man, pointing his cardboard sign our way.

"It's the Channel 5 cameraman... they're leaving!"

In retrospect, our little threesome would have been less conspicuous had we all huddled under an umbrella and cloaked ourselves in black leather capes. And it didn't help that my big Ford was so radiantly red.

The placard and banner crowd, along with the outdoor concessions trailer line, all immediately emptied in our direction. They were closely followed by scramblers from the propane-heated tent, then joined by others who poured out from the hospital lobby. News traveled at the speed of sight.

Fighting panic, I flung open the nearest door and shoved Freak and the camera into the second seat. Saundra piled in on the front passenger side, frantically urging me on.

By the time I had the SUV in gear, it was already too late.

A more reckless man might have tossed the dice and gunned it. If there had only been a couple of photographers running straight into my grill, I might have risked playing chicken myself. Instead, three dozen or more reporters were recording my face and license plates before I even started to roll. I managed to drive a quick couple of car lengths, then was forced to slow, then was barely able to advance. Some of these folks were apparently prepared to die for our story.

As a teenager, I'd accidentally bumped over a neighbor's cat. The feeling of the little crunching lurch, and the drama that followed, had left me sick. I supposed it might be almost that bad if I rolled over one of these.

I continued to inch forward as best I could, parting the seas up the bottlenecked drive for another ten yards before finally slogging to a complete stop, scarcely the length of a field goal kick from the open road.

"They've got Freak," someone yelled.

On reflex, I double-checked my locks for the third time.

Reporters thronged in from every direction. A man wearing thick black glasses and a white robe forced his way to the front of my rig, clearing a path with jabs and wild swings with a sign declaring, as best I could tell: "Hell No, We Won't Go!" Whatever that was supposed to mean.

Mouths steamed, faces pressed, and greasy hands streaked nimbus smudges around my windows. Heavy jackets and sharp zippers scratched my paint from every side.

As I thought about it later, I could hardly blame them. Other than Saundra's two news clips, the world had not gotten any good looks at the Reverend Bill Jacobs since before his fall. Competing media venues from around the world were frustrated by having to buy the same tired shots over and over off the wire, all billed through High-5-at Five News. Major players and young wannabes alike were hungry, starved for fresh material of their own. Travel expenses needed to be justified, and so far, they had nada to share but a frozen brick hospital backdrop for their endless talking head commentaries that rambled each hour with nothing new to ever say.

And here he was: Freak in the flesh. Close enough to touch. Even the shot of a dark nose in the shadows of a drawn orange hood was better than anything they'd gotten so far.

"He's in there all right," shouted a woman. "In the back seat!" cried another.

Saundra quietly turned pale, shaking her head. I bothered to wonder how she felt about being trapped on this side of the lens for once, but thought better of asking. Over my shoulder, Freak sank low, buried within his hood. He'd gone back to praying or cursing, and he was shaking hard. I started really feeling sorry for the guy. Started getting angry.

A man from Texas, judging from his fur coat, climbed onto my rig's push bar for a better angle through the front window. Emboldened, two more quickly followed. Not to be outdone, a bearded young man in a blue stocking cap began crawling across my hood, not stopping until his wide-angle lens was snug against my windshield, inches from my mounting fury.

I flashed a fist, then thought to reach down to my controls. The first squirt of wiper fluid caught him off guard, and the swinging wiper blade nearly knocked the camera from his hand. By the third squirt, his eyes were stinging, and he gave me some room to breathe.

I put the rig in neutral, revved the engine as threateningly as possible, then laid on the horn. For a moment, it worked. Especially in front and on the hood, folks began moving back. I slipped it into gear and started to inch though the pack.

Then some wild paparazzi opportunist—in a surge of inspiration or vertigo—knocked over the nearest Porta-Potty. Thankfully, nobody was inside at the time. At least, nobody was coming out. Either way, there it was, barricading the exit and oozing across my path.

Folks cleared out from around the pooling filth, and I suddenly caught sight of a possible escape. My mind flashed to what an Expedition's push bar could do to anything as portable as a fibreglass outhouse. I geared down to 4-Low and fed my beastie a surge of fuel.

We headed for the gap in the crowd where the butt end of the potty met the snowbank, figuring to push through at a whopping 5 mph, engine in a roar, horn on fire.

At ten miles per hour, we might have made it. As it was, by the time we crawled screaming up to the spilt potty in 4-Low, angry camera folk had already taken all the higher ground. It became an ambush.

A rout.

Hemmed in, I had to stop. Hostiles shot down at us from the plowed snowbanks on every side. They were falling all over themselves and each other, surefooted one moment, then arms flailing, and then slipping, sinking or spilling sideways the next. There was no way to break through the snowbanks without risking the loss of life or limb. I weighed the consequences.

Meanwhile, the growing mob behind barred any hope of retreat. As for pushing through the roadblock ahead... cameramen were already violating the prone Porta-Potty itself, mounting its side, securing their holds, and zooming their lenses straight down through my windshield. Relentlessly, they probed my cab for any hints of Freak.

I turned to Saundra. "I'm going to play some music. You okay with Sadcore Rock?"

She shrugged. "This is insane. Who do these people think they are?"

"Reporters," I said. "Hustling for Emmys, I suppose."

"I'm calling 911."

"Whatever," I grumbled.

"Do something," she snapped, yanking out her stylus and scratching a quick note onto her phone.

"Yes sir, lady. You say frog, I jump." I winced in a camera flash. "By the way, how's that 911 going?"

I reached for a CD.

"Hey, back there," I called over my shoulder, as sympathetically as I could manage. "Are you okay?"

Freak looked up for a moment, briefly connecting with my gaze.

"It's not your fault," he said.

"Sure it is. It always is."

"No," he sighed, despondent, retreating back into his earflaps and hood. "We should have prayed."

I inserted the CD, cranked the volume, then closed my eyes and waited for the cavalry.

SECURED

"Let's just say that I work for the Department of Homeland Security."

Freak nodded, willing to let it go at that. Rainbow tassels from his wonky hat swayed near his mouth, but he made no attempt to brush them aside or remove the cap.

"And I believe," said the dark suit, turning to me, "that you've already met Deputy Sheriff Andy Dekkers?" He motioned to my whiskered watchdog in the dark uniform from the hospital.

"Yes," I smiled, faking it, reaching to shake the sheriff's hand. "Andy and I are actually quite close. We did a sleepover."

Agent Wilcox, gave me an odd look.

"Ignore him," sighed the sheriff. "He's like that."

"By the way, Andy," I said, rigorously shaking his fist. "I really liked your cop show when I was a kid. I loved all those after-school reruns on channel 91. You and Barney Fife... what a team."

"Hilarious." He shook his head and tugged his black mustache. "I'm surprised that I've never heard that before."

"Come on," I called, sweeping the room, trying to unwind. "Lighten up, everybody. Let's all take a load off and talk this through." I motioned toward the mammoth sectional and headed towards the bar. "Drink... anyone?"

Steve was already at the counter, lifting the linen napkin and rifling the basket for pastries left behind from our breakfast cart. Freak carefully hung the orange parka on one of the pegs inside the front closet door, adjusted his earflap a little more to the left, then drifted towards a chair. Saundra remained planted at the door.

"Agent Wilcox," she fumed. "I'm going to have to insist that you allow Steve to go back down to retrieve our equipment from Mark's car."

"Hey," I shouted from beside the wine rack. "Call it a truck. Or call it a rig. But please, Saundra... my red beastie is *never* to be called a car."

"A beastie," she glared, "would have gotten us out of there. Your car whimpered like a scared little kitten."

Hmm. Forget the wine. This called for a whiskey sour.

"Help me out here, Sheriff Dekker." I opened the cabinet and found the bar's stash of hard liquor shooters. "Andy, in your professional opinion—as one who has sworn an oath to law and order—is it better to drive *around* journalists... or *over* them?"

"Cruel," laughed Steve. "That could have been me under your fender."

"The reporters would have moved," she fumed.

"Sure," I said, selecting a couple favorites from the little rows of familiar labels. "Just like you would have stepped aside, right, Saundra? With the story of the year sitting right there three feet away...."

"Enough," barked Freak. "You two can finish your nonsense later." He turned to the tall stranger in a tie. "Agent Wilcox, Saundra deserves an answer. Why did you insist that she leave their equipment in Mark's car?"

"Rig!" I corrected. "It's *not* a car. Never was, never will be. Show some respect." I pulled several square glasses from the shelf and began dropping in some ice.

"Water for me," said Wilcox. "Same for Sheriff Dekkers." He turned to Saundra and Freak. "Sorry. First we need to talk. Then I will have someone bring up the rest of your things... once you know the rules."

"Beer works for me," said Steve, crumbs already on his shirt, reaching for his second Danish.

Saundra stepped toward the agent. "Seriously. We need our things. Now."

"Soon," he said, forcing a Teflon smile. "As I said, first, we need to establish the ground rules."

"Not without my camera...."

"Listen," frowned Andy, his hand absently resting on his holster. "You reporters don't always get to call the shots. Especially when you're into something that's way over your heads. You've got no idea what is going on right now. If we hadn't been nearby to save your hides...."

"You sure took your time about it...."

"Seats!" I bellowed. The Earth didn't move, but at least they shut up.

"Please," I said, filling two glasses from the tap. "Would everybody please just sit down. You're all making me nervous. Especially Andy Griffith over there with his hand on his gun." Andy caught himself and quickly dropped his hand to his side. "Why don't you all talk about the weather for a few minutes and let me make my drink."

They reluctantly started moving towards the big couch and overstuffed chairs. But then Wilcox peeled wide and strode over to the soaring bank of thick windows facing the ski lifts and dark pines to the west. I glanced his way. Beyond our balcony rail, the slopes were surprisingly open. Folks were probably maxing out their credit cards. Packing down the hill for cheaper motels. Maybe hoping to wait things out in Denver until the airlines were up again and could fly them back to their homes and jobs and schools in other states.

Wilcox studied the lay of the mountain, surveying the condos and lodges nearby. He stood there plenty long enough to make me nervous.

"Hey, Wilcox," I said. "Wrong direction. Too much shade." I pointed the other way. "The spring break bikini skiers are usually sunning themselves on Duke's Run this time of day."

When he failed to reply, I volunteered, "The lodge has provided complimentary binoculars. They're hanging over there by the front door." When he still said nothing, I added, "So... are you scouting for snipers, or what?"

He responded by stepping to the edge of the windowed wall and reaching into the heavy jade drapes. In smooth easy draws, he pulled the cords until our living room view was entirely veiled. Light streamed through the massive upper panes on the loft level, but our privacy had been secured on the lower level of the main room.

Wilcox pulled a wooden stool from the bar and positioned a throne for himself at the head of the living room circle. He eyeballed his subjects down his nose, sitting strategically higher than the couch and the two matching leather chairs. He abruptly pivoted his focus to me behind the bar.

"Care to join us?" he demanded.

"So..." I retorted, making him wait, leaning into the dark granite countertop. "I guess you figure it's now *your* party, huh?"

"It *is* my party... as long as I'm picking up the tab."

True, as it turned out, we were all technically staying at the lodge as his guests. Or as guests of his agency. And, also true, if not for his help, Freak, Saundra and I might still be squirming like bugs under a glass in the hospital parking lot.

But nobody likes to have his face rubbed in it.

"Fine, Wilcox. If it's your party, then you can do the dishes when we leave."

I scooped up the two waters and marched to Sheriff Andy first. "Ice, right? Lots of ice?" Next, I handed Wilcox his. I stomped back to the bar, then hefted the nearest pine stool. I carried it to the fireplace end of the ring, dropped it with a heavy thump opposite of Wilcox, then climbed aboard.

"Aye, captain," I smirked. "Present and accounted for. Commence with the floggings."

Wilcox slowly heaved his chest, unblinking. Measuring me. Weighing each of us in turn. Saundra continued to glare, her legs tightly crossed from her ankles all the way to her hips. Steve held the pastry basket in his lap, looking back to the bar as if cheated out of something sweet and bubbly to rinse the berry from his teeth. Freak sat beneath his elephant flaps, stone faced, his scars all but lost in shadows.

"Okay," said Wilcox at last. He shrugged in surrender.

"Mr. Hanson, you go finish making your drink. Get the cameraman his beer. Find out whatever it is that Ms. Paige needs to relax." Wilcox looked back at me and grinned. "But no pot. I know it's legal here in Colorado, but if you pull out the weed, then we gotta leave." He stuck a finger in his collar and loosened his tie. "And despite what you think right now, you really don't want us to leave. Trust me."

He turned to Andy. "Take off your jacket and call down to the team. Have one of your men bring up the lady's gear."

As luck would have it, Wilcox was Rocky Mountain born and raised. He'd lived on military and intelligence assignments for a couple of decades, but it only took one five minute head-butting exchange in the lee of a hewn-rock fireplace for common sense and practical courtesies to return. A heavy hand comes up frostbit anywhere above 6,000 feet. In a land where the sun rises over sage-blown cowboy flats and settles behind jagged untamed peaks, back-East style silk ties and snobbery incite more scorn than respect. He unbuttoned in a hurry, once he remembered the terrain.

"Sorry," he said for the second time. "I know it's your station's property, Saundra. I know you have a job to do." He took a sip from his water. "And you're damn good at it, from what I've seen."

"Thank you," she smiled, finally restored to her radiant self. "I'm glad you understand." She patted the closed equipment bag at her feet, then stroked the black bundle like it was a favored puppy. "I'll leave it packed for now. I know you've got a job to do, just like me."

"Wilcox," I added, tipping from my third drink, "thanks for coming down off that high stool of yours. And it was mighty neighborly of you to take off your tie."

The agent touched a finger to his open white collar.

I smiled. "The last time I saw a neck leash in Summit County was at my grandpa's funeral. Not looped around the preacher's neck, mind you, but on my dead Pappy Joe... starched stiff there in the box. He's buried not far from here. He bought his one-and-only necktie mail order, back in the fifties. Said he'd need it one day. Sure enough, one day... he finally did." I raised my drink in a toast. "Wilcox, may you never need your tie again. At least not for another week."

He laughed. "I get it. Sorry I came on so thick-headed up front. But we do need to talk. If they put me in a pine box next week, they'll probably be planting us all the same day. There's some serious stuff going down in the world right now. Even here in Summit County."

Freak leaned forward from the opposite chair. "We will respect the fact you cannot tell us everything," he said. Tassels from his left flap swayed slightly with the movement of his jaw. "But it's time to put everything on the table that you can." He leaned back and closed his eyes. "I suspect my survival is creating... issues."

"No offense," chimed Andy, "but, hell yes. My job would be whole a lot easier right now if you'd blown up with the rest of them."

Wilcox lifted an eyebrow in Andy's direction, but he did not attempt to rein the man in.

"Why, Andy," I chuckled, "I'm surprised at you."

"I'm just saying," the sheriff continued, "everybody is on mandatory overtime. Not just us, but first responders in every department from here to Denver. Personnel are being shuffled left and right, and outside guys like Agent Wilcox—good guys, mostly—are giving all the orders." He looked at Wilcox. "I'm not complaining, mind you. But it sucks."

I glanced at the empty glass in Andy's hands, wondering if I'd somehow filled it with gin by mistake.

"Thanks, Andy," said Wilcox. "I appreciate your honesty. Everyone has been under a lot of pressure. You've been excellent to work with, and I hope you'll hang in there with me. It is extremely helpful for me to have someone at my side who knows the lay of the land the way you do."

Andy nodded, smoothing a crease from his side-striped trousers, satisfied he'd been heard.

"Reverend Jacobs," continued Wilcox. "I agree. You need to know what's going on."

"Please," he insisted. "I know it's hard, but you're going to have to call me Freak."

"Okay then. Freak." Wilcox shifted in his seat. "Yes, your survival has complicated things."

"What kind of things?" asked Saundra, clearly preparing to take mental notes.

"Saundra," said Wilcox, "I respect you enough to not be speaking around you 'off the record.' Some of what I share will seem so important that you will feel like it's your obligation to communicate this information to your superiors, as well as with your viewing public. All I'm asking is that you think carefully about what you put on the air, and that you respect how I am forced to withhold certain pieces of sensitive information. Acceptable?"

"Understood." A black and silver stylus materialized in Saundra's right hand. "With what you've said in mind, I'm willing to leave the camera packed for now. But I'd like to be able to take notes." A fresh screen was already glowing from her phone. "Acceptable?"

He smiled. "I would expect no less. Whatever you decide to air, at minimum, it should be accurate." He turned to Freak. "How about you? Are you good with Saundra's presence as a reporter? Or do you need to come to some kind of agreement with her as well?"

Freak shrugged. "I'm not sure. We might have to talk this through again when she pulls out the camera. I do trust Saundra. Anything I say can be quoted. But I'm not clear yet where I stand on the images."

"Understood," she smiled. "I cannot speak for the other stations and networks. Based upon what happened in the parking lot today, they're going to film whatever they can get away with. You and the Falling Skies Massacre are still the biggest stories in the world right now. But what I *can* promise is that Channel 5 will treat you with respect. We will honor your requests about any footage that we air. Freak, the more that you and I can work together on this, the more it's a win-win for both sides."

"Both sides?" he grinned.

"For everyone," she smiled back, jotting her first note.

CONSPIRACIES

Saundra buried herself in her note app.

She looked up from her frantic scribbling only occasionally, checking an expression, tapping the stylus to her lips while clarifying an uncertain point. Wilcox spent the next 20 minutes reviewing what he could, bringing us all up to speed.

Wilcox There were several theories about how the terrorists managed to coordinate and pull off such a complicated attack on a global scale. Each scenario was more frightening than the last. All of them involved insiders receiving huge payoffs, or worse, insiders who were committed to the cause.

Wilcox was one of a dozen special agents dispatched to the four American crash sites. All carried high-level security clearances and direct access to intelligence and resources he could not discuss. His task was the most clear-cut of their four assignments. But his was also the most difficult. His mission was, quite simply: Freak.

Our fiasco trying to sneak Freak from the hospital was a personal embarrassment. We'd beaten Wilcox by less than an hour from having his operation fully in place. Even while we were faking our sobbing exit through the ER, Wilcox was briefing his team and positioning his people so that at no time would Freak be able to move anywhere without observation cover and a protective escort.

"Protective?" asked Steve.

"Of course," blurted Freak, looking around the room. "They want me dead."

"Who wants you dead?" I asked.

"For one," said Wilcox, "the terrorists. Freak's survival represents unfinished business. As long as he walks, there are questions about whether Allah is really all-powerful. Every time Freak appears on the air and mentions he has been hearing messages from Jesus and that he is under divine protection, the world is forced to wonder whether the terrorist's really have God on their side."

"On the other hand," said Andy, "now that Freak is on the world's stage, if they *can* assassinate him, then terrorists would be striking a huge psychological blow. Almost like scoring two shocking attacks for the price of one."

"Right," said Wilcox. "Possibly with minimal effort... and relatively minimal expense."

"Minimal expense?" Saundra glanced up from her notes.

"A hired assassin," sighed Freak. "Or maybe an open contract. They wouldn't even need to kill me themselves."

Steve nearly dropped his beer. "Are you saying someone is going to get paid for killing Freak?"

"I can neither confirm nor deny that sort of claim." Wilcox blinked at Saundra's frozen S Pen. "But, logically speaking, such a contract would make a lot of sense."

"The drapes?" I said.

"Right. It's probably in the interest of everyone in this room for the drapes remain closed. Also, that nobody comes or goes without first working out a plan with me and Andy. I've got several more men nearby on this assignment, and Andy has the rest of the local team at his disposal. We're not holding you as prisoners or trying to make things hard on you, but you need to know what we're all up against. The danger is real."

Hmm. "Who else?" I asked at last. "Wilcox, when Freak said folks want him dead, you said, 'For one... the terrorists.' That kinda sounds like you've got a list?"

He studied me, making no attempt to answer.

"I assume," I added, "that you've got bigger threats in mind than the rioting Kentucky frat boys who blame Freak for derailing the NCAA March Madness playoffs?"

"Right," said Steve. "Who else is on the not-a-fan-of-Freak list?"

"For another," ventured Saundra, "the list has got to include some pretty powerful movers and shakers from high places on the home front. I can imagine a number of politicians and business interests who have a lot on the line right now. Even if they're not killers themselves, they probably owe it to their constituencies and stake holders to run a cost-benefit analysis on Freak's life."

"What do you mean?" I asked.

"You should have heard," said Steve, "some of our discussions in the production truck. Heated calls were coming in from all directions, up and down the line of command. All the way to the top of the network. Maybe even from beyond the network."

"Mark," said Saundra, "think about it."

"Advertisers?"

"Of course. Do the math. Let's say you sell expensive automobiles. Freak comes on the air and prophesies that millions of people are going to die. That's bad enough. But what if something actually does happen, a disaster fitting what Freak described?"

Saundra glanced at Freak, then continued. "So Freak gets back on the air a week after one of his predictions seems to come true. Now millions of people are starting to take him seriously as a reliable prophet. Then he says God is really going to bring the hammer down once and for all. This time he says God told him the world will end next October. How do you think that's going to impact the stability of our society... let alone automobile sales?"

The room fell deathly quiet.

"I'd buy one," I grinned at last. "I wouldn't make any payments, but I'd be out there the next day, cruising showrooms for a red Shelby Raptor. If the world's going down, then more than ever, a guy should try to have a good last ride. A ride to end all rides. Why not?"

Saundra shook her head. "Schoolboys aside, the impact could be devastating. Automobiles, boats, gold watches... you name it."

Wilcox decided to complete the scenario. "You name it... is right. Not just luxury items, but all sorts of durable goods and industries could be devastated. Everything from carpet stores to roofing crews. From furniture manufacturing to the ship yards. Who would be spending money on those things? Even a twenty-percent drop in orders will typically shut down a lot of big factories for a month or more. Who would be left showing up for work?"

"Who would bother to pay their taxes?" I added, the picture snapping into focus. "Or who would even bother to go to school... especially if their teachers were staying home anyway?"

"But," said Freak, "the Lord saved me. I was snatched from certain death. I was rescued for a reason."

"To destroy the world's economy?" Asked Wilcox. "To create chaos in the streets? Is that your goal?"

"Of course not. But the Lord has saved me to be a prophet for the end times. It is imperative that I hear from God and find more clarity on this. I've got to boldly warn the world...."

"You see," sighed the agent, "This is exactly the kind of inflammatory talk capable of turning society upside down. Reverend Jacobs, and a hundred like him, have been preaching Armageddon for decades. Maybe from the beginning of time. Interesting, perhaps, but seldom taken too seriously by the general population in the modern West."

"Until now," I said.

"Exactly," said Wilcox. "Until this week. Until one of those preachers got blown from the sky... and lived to preach another day. More wild-eyed than ever. Insisting he was saved by angels with a message from God."

"I was," said Freak, his voice matter-of-fact.

"Of course you were. What kind of apocalypse would it be if we didn't have clouds swirling with thousands of angels?"

"The sky," said Freak, "was clear. No clouds. And only two angels."

"My boss," said Saundra, "has been texting me some viewer stats and survey numbers. "The public, and I don't mean just the hysterical fringe, they all want to hear what Freak has to say. Folks are making bets around the water cooler. They might not agree with Freak, but they want to hear more from him. All kinds of weird stuff is starting to go viral....millions of hits on absurd sites making wild speculations about what Freak will say is going to happen next."

Hmm. "So you're saying that as much as the terrorists might want to shut Freak up, perhaps certain folks in government and business might...."

"Let's not get ahead of ourselves," said Wilcox. "That's pure conjecture. Paranoia, even."

"There are others," said Freak. "The list includes powerful others who you have not yet thought to name."

His voice was low, as somber as I'd ever heard it.

"There are those who want me dead even more than anyone you've thought yet to name."

"Who?" asked Saundra.

"Thousands of religious fanatics and cult members... from both the right and the left. And even more than those unstable masses, the strategic forces that have tremendous influence and strongholds within their ranks."

"Their leaders?" asked Steve.

"No. I am speaking about the real powers behind the men and women in these groups... the demons."

Well, that opened a can of worms. I figured Steve could use another beer, and I sure as heck needed to uncap a couple more shooters. I fetched Saundra a glass of Merlot and tried to stay out of the fray, especially when I realized which side she was on. As a kid, Saundra must have done some serious time in Sunday school, because she was tracking pretty close with Freak, and she hardly ever disagreed with him about any of it. Steve and Andy, on the other hand, would not give an inch. A conversation that started fairly academic quickly spiked into sensationalism, maybe even sport.

From the sidelines, the entertainment value of the contest was considerable. Beauty and the Beast vs. the equally unlikely duo of Rumpled Plaid and Pressed Pleats. I kept the drinks flowing, while Wilcox mostly sat tight lipped, barely shaking his head yes or no, depending upon the volley.

Finally, I insisted that we order some dinner. By then, we couldn't even agree on pizza toppings, so I called down to the kitchen for a small buffet, a little of everything. Plus a couple more bottles of red and white to plug the holes that had shown up in the wine rack.

When the food arrived, I finally found a chance to score points with Saundra by making myself busy in the dining area, setting the table with one hand, sipping a crisp Riesling with the other. The massive pine table could seat ten, so I put a little extra space between the plates and slid a couple of the chairs off into a corner. I poured wine and waters for every seat, found some fancy silverware and napkins, and called it good.

"Let's eat," I shouted into the din. Five minutes later, we'd figured it out. Saundra was next to me on one side, Steve and Andy sat at the other.

The big guns positioned themselves at the head and the foot of the table. One held sway with full government authority and a ridiculously stiff collar, the other with a silly hat and head full of ancient Bible. I'm pretty confident none of us were certain which end held the most power.

"Thanks," said Wilcox, turning to me. "I appreciate you taking care of these arrangements."

"No problem," I said, raising my glass. "It's my pleasure... as long as you keep picking up the tab."

"I hope," said Freak, "that nobody will mind if I pray?"

One or two of us might have shrugged a mite, but Freak didn't seem to notice. Maybe more of us would have put up a fuss if we'd realized where he was going with it.

"Oh, Lord," he began, softly, in a churchy-singy way, "have mercy on we who have gathered here around this bounteous table...."

He lost me right away, and since I was looking down already, I decided to sneak a gander at Saundra's leg. Hmm. The lamb on our cart had nothing on that thigh. About the time my gaze started getting a bit more aggressive, something Freak said caught my ear.

"... and we know that our Savior who is *within* us... he is greater than the Evil One, the dark enemy who prowls the darkness *around* us...."

Hmm. How'd we get off from the food cart to this devil talk and Holy Ghost warfare stuff so quickly again?

"And, Lord, I'm asking for our safety. Not just for your prophet, but for those you've called to protect and bear witness to the work of your prophet. Protection, too, for my wife and children, and for the families of those...." his voice trailed off.

There we sat, waiting for an amen. For something. Anything. I glanced across to Steve, whose hands were awkwardly folded, but whose eyes were now as open as mine. Then Wilcox, then Andy. For a journalist, Saundra was surprisingly patient. When it got to be just her and Freak, I started wracking my brain for a clever toast; I figured a pithy salute might serve as good as anything for a make-do amen. One came to mind. I rehearsed it twice, then cleared my throat to begin.

"Thank you, Lord," whispered Freak, beating me to the punch. "Amen."

"Amen," echoed Saundra.

"Amen," chorused a tenor and a bass.

"That was lovely," I said. "Thank you, Pastor Freak. And now, for your dining pleasure tonight we have...."

"Wait," interrupted Freak.

Hmm. "Yes?"

"I have an announcement."

Of course.

"The Lord has instructed me to remove my hat at the table."

And the good news is?

"Not just for this meal, but perhaps from now on. I'm to have more courage. Not to cower behind these flaps in shame."

"Are you sure about this?" stammered Wilcox. "You'll stand out like a sore thumb wherever you go. You'll be a sitting duck. And that means we'll all be exposed."

"We'll be safe." Freak pushed back his chair and took a deep breath. "At least for tonight," he smiled, "we are fully covered where it counts the most."

He slowly reached up. Gently, he lifted the absurd sherpa cap, as if removing the crown from a dying king.

Before us, obliging us to gawk, compelling us to turn away, glowed Freak's scarred face. Unchanged from the other day.

In all its glory.

In all its horror.

He handed the hat back to Steve. "Here," he said. "Thanks. But I won't be using this anymore."

"No, keep it," sputtered Steve. "Just in case...."

"You are kind," said Freak. "But I insist." He dropped the hat past the table into Steve's reluctant lap.

"Freak," I asked. "What's going on?"

"It's going to be okay, Mark. God is with us."

There was a confidence in his voice that I'd not heard since his global interview, since his conversation with Saundra where he'd declared to the world that millions more would die.

"Freak," I protested, suddenly feeling far too dry for all the booze I'd swallowed in the last hour. "You're scaring me again."

"There's nothing to fear, Mark. I know what I'm doing."

Another monstrous military helicopter thumped low at the distant end of the valley. It hovered for a few moments, then swooped up over a ridge and faded away.

"Our security," said Wilcox, "is tighter than you might think. And we're beefing it up more tonight. But I still think...."

"Mark," said Freak, ignoring Wilcox. "Fear not, for the Lord is our strength and shield. We are safe. We shall all sleep well. We shall remain under His special protection throughout the night."

"How do you know?" I insisted.

"Do you remember how I told you that angels were with me? That angels were singing over me as I fell from the plane?"

"Yes."

"Well..." he said, a wry smile forming on his lips. "Look around. If you have eyes to see... they're back. The angels returned while we sat in prayer."

Saundra gasped.

She turned from one side of the room to the other.

"Yes," she whispered, excitedly. Fearfully. "One at the windows. The other at the door."

She closed her eyes. Opened them again and beamed both ways.

"And they're huge!"

16
MORNING'S LIGHT

I didn't see any angels.

Not that night. Never did. Never will.

I suppose the power of suggestion is a dangerous force, and it takes a sharp and determined intellect to resist its snares.

In the morning, reason again prevailed. After a good night's rest, Saundra regained her senses. When pressed, she doubted herself whether angels had really appeared.

It had been a delicious—but awkward—feast after Freak's prayer. She'd blinked a few times, then said they were gone.

Then we moved some furniture around and channel surfed the news on the big screen in the living room. From time to time, one of us would appear in a story. Steve and I tried to elevate the mood with occasional irreverent editorial observations.

The Colorado disaster news footage was comprised mostly of wobbled handheld shots of fallen debris, along with repeats of Freak's statements from previous Channel 5 clips. Sometimes a few frames of chaos were spliced into a story from our episode in the hospital parking lot, including a very flattering shot of me shaking my fist through my red beastie's windshield. The whacko protesters made for good additional local color, and at one point a camera zoomed in on the "Hell No, We Won't Go" sign. Unfortunately, the reporter failed to further investigate or interpret the sign, thus leaving me and the rest of the world in bewildered suspense.

As disturbing as it all was, we only lasted an hour or so in front of the TV. On the economic front, Wall Street and almost every market but precious metals took another day of hammering. Pockets of civil unrest were breaking out even in unlikely places.

It was all too much.

Exhausted, we snuffed the news. We each made our way to our own rooms, ready to hunker down, spent from conversation and all of the unsettling reports of angels and mayhem.

Wilcox and Andy had their guys bring luggage and equipment up from their rig. They commandeered the game room for their office and shared the big room downstairs with the two queen beds for their sleeping.

Freak took the other double room in the loft, and Steve slept on his favorite wing of the couch, this time adding bedding from the sidebar drawer. Saundra and I stuck with the master suites that we'd already claimed, her up and me down.

As I said, in the morning, things were making sense again. Freak was showering in the common bathroom below, and I had drifted to the upstairs loft lounge, in a chair at Saundra's side.

"Nerves," she confessed. "Every once in a while, I just lose it. For a professionally trained journalist, it's kind of embarrassing."

Today, Saundra was smudge free. She had showered, finished her makeup, and dressed for the camera before leaving her room. I'd brought up a healthy continental breakfast from the cart, and I was pouring Mimosas when she finally presented herself for popular consumption. We chatted and chewed on the right light stuff, then ventured into the unknown.

"You sure seemed to be convinced at the time," I said.

"So," she asked demurely, "I seemed to really believe I was seeing something, huh?"

"You said they were huge."

"Two of them, right?"

"That's what you said. But I knew better. I squinted high and low, and there definitely were *not* two angels." I nodded and winked. "Just the one."

She smiled.

"All the same," I added, "I am curious. Can you remember what you *thought* you saw?"

Saundra looked away, down from the loft to the drapes below.

"It's strange," she said. She extended her hand for a cluster of grapes. "I can hardly even describe them. It was like I knew they were there, I could see them, but... I couldn't see them. And then they were gone."

Steve clodded up the stairs along the rail, still wearing his new white robe, a mug of coffee steaming from his free hand.

"Are you swapping angel tales?" he asked, throwing himself onto the opposite corner of the sectional. "I wanna hear this."

"It's silly," she mumbled. "Let's forget it."

"No," insisted Steve. "This is a heck of a story. Last night, you were pretty emphatic. I wish I'd had the camera rolling. Who knows?" He leaned over for an apple, then chomped down in an overloud crunch. "High 5 at Five...." he laughed. "All the latest news... and your best source for everything you need to know about spirits that go bump in the night."

"Denver's A-Team," I added, "for those who will settle for nothing but the best in apocalyptic Devil-Busters."

Saundra started to rise.

"Steve's right," I said, motioning for her to sit back down. "This is interesting. What sort of ghost does the mind summon while under the spell of the Reverend Freak?"

She was standing now, looking down at me, uncertain whether to grow defensive or to play along. Her professional side prevailed, and she committed to put an end to the discussion once and for all.

"If you must know," she said with a grin, "the figure by the window glimmered, brightly, but not harshly. He emitted a sense of warmth." She glanced toward the drapes. "He was shimmering in some sort of frightful, pulsing energy... and yet, it was as if he was smiling at me."

"Of course he was happy to look at you. He had eyes, right?"

"The other one, the darker apparition at the door, he looked all business. Stern. Even mean."

"He? You know it was a male?"

"That was the feeling I got."

"Did the guy by the door have long hair, or short?" I asked.

"Hair? I'm not sure. Short, I guess."

"A beard?"

"Maybe."

"Good grief," I laughed. "It was my Pappy Joe, back from the grave!"

Saundra grinned, then tossed her last grape at my head. I caught it in my mouth.

"I warned my Uncle Ed," I complained, "I told him that he hadn't dug that hole deep enough."

Saundra shook her head and sat back down on the spot where I patted the couch.

"Let's forget about it," she said. "Today, I can see that I imagined the whole thing." She flashed a coy smile at Steve. "I'd really rather this silly drunken episode didn't make the rounds."

"So that's it," snickered Steve. "Censorship, eh? No angel story after all?"

"I guess not," said Saundra. "Sorry for the false lead. I guess it was all the wine... and those dark drapes. My eyes were probably making fuzzy spots after squeezing so long during Freak's rambling prayer."

"Retraction accepted," said Steve. He rose and headed back for the stairs. "Although, in truth, I'd kinda prefer believing it was angels rather than illusions. Wilcox put a little scare into me last night. I'm not too keen about being glued to a guy with a contract on his head."

"More fantasies," I said. "Conspiracy theories. Trumped up nonsense just to create job security for the feds."

"Sure," he said, heading down the stairs. "I'm going to take a shower and check up on my gear. You never know when one of those fantasies might come dropping from the clouds or flying through a window. I suppose I'd better be ready just in case."

"I'll join you in a few minutes," called Saundra. "Boss says we've got to give him something good today, or he'll put Tom Jackson on the assignment." She laughed. "As if."

"As if!" he called back from half way down the flight. "Should I wear boots or sneakers today? Let me know what's up once you've made a plan."

"Mark and I will be right down." She turned back to me. "It's settled, then. No more talk about angels. But we do need to discuss what's next with Freak."

"I'm all ears."

"Well, in the hospital, he referred to you as his witness. Unless he's changed his mind about you, that probably means he's hoping you'll stick with him for a while."

"I suppose. I guess we're a team. Me and Freak... and Wilcox and Andy."

"And me?" She batted her eyes. "Do I get to tag along? Do I get to spend another night here with you in the lodge?"

"Are you playing me?"

"Of course I'm playing you," she laughed. "I'm a professional. Anything for a story."

"Anything?"

"Well, not that!"

"Shucks. And I almost thought we had a deal."

She swatted me with a pillow from the couch.

"Foul," I cried. "If you're going to start coming at me with your pillow charms, I don't stand a chance." I pulled the embroidered pillow from her hands and placed it on my lap. "You know all the tricks of the trade, don't you, Saundra?"

"My daddy was a contractor. He said construction workers must learn how to position their hands on a sheet of plywood, and then they've got to bend their knees so they can lift with their legs. If they don't, they'll wreck their backs and lose their jobs." Saundra giggled. "Since I don't want to lose my job, I guess I've learned to use my legs."

"You're a professional, all right. A professional flirt."

"Yes" she said, tugging the pillow from my lap. "Of course I know how to grab... and when to flip my hair." She tossed her head. A stunning blond strand caught in an alluring wisp behind her ear. "It's all part of the job."

"A sheet of plywood, huh? That's how you see me? Lots of splinters, I suppose?"

"Maybe," she teased.

"Well, okay then. Since it's all part of the job, I'm game." I swung around and stretched out on the couch. "Go ahead."

"Go ahead and what...?"

"Lift me with your legs."

17 BOSSES

Saundra could move me, but the day's ambitious agenda did not include lifting me with her legs.

By 9:30 AM, she somehow had gathered all hands on deck, fed and dressed, reluctantly assembled for a family parley. Freak and Wilcox established the bow and stern from the armed chairs, while the rest of us dutifully inclined or reclined on the sectional. Except for Steve, who intermittently padded back and forth replenishing rations from the galley.

"What I am saying," she insisted, "is that it's time for a plan."

"Your plan..." queried Andy, "or Reverend Jacob's plan?"

"Freak," corrected Freak.

"I don't see why both plans can't be the same." Saundra turned from Andy's taut dark uniform to the white collared and re-tied Agent Wilcox. "You said that we weren't prisoners. You only asked that we keep informed."

"Actually," he corrected, "what I said was that we are facing significant dangers here. I said nobody should come or go without a coordinated protective escort, as well as a thoroughly developed set of contingencies. With everything drawn up and cleared through my team."

"My goodness," sniped Saundra. "That part must have flown clear over my silly little head. What I thought I heard yesterday was that your security team was watching out for our safety. I don't recall anything about 'sets of contingencies' having to be 'drawn up and cleared.'"

Saundra glanced to her cameraman for support. All she caught was his ear; Steve was hunched at the countertop taking an inventory of the remaining pastries.

"Agent Wilcox," she said, readjusting her sights. "You mentioned nothing last night about taking authority over how we should do our jobs."

"I'm not telling you how to do your jobs. But we cannot afford a repeat of yesterday's debacle at the hospital. Which, I might add, drew the wrath of my superiors. It is essential from now on...."

"Please," said Freak. "I'm a little confused here. You two keep talking about doing your jobs. What about me?"

We all looked at him. As long as we could. Those aft of Freak's scars blinked away first. Sleep hadn't facilitated any noticeable improvements. If anything, the gouged tissue flamed more brightly in the wake of a night's worth of pillow pressing. Then again, maybe the steam shower was to blame.

"Okay," said Saundra, politely addressing Freak's right shoulder. "I'm sorry. But as you can imagine, the station is screaming for another interview. Or at least to provide a substantive update...."

"I understand," said Freak.

"This is not just for the Channel 5 Denver market, but for the entire world. Everybody...."

"I understand," repeated Freak.

"And yesterday, when we came and got you from the hospital, you insinuated that when we got back to the lodge...." She glanced at me, then back to Freak. "When Mark offered to come get you, I'm certain he, like me, was under the impression...."

"*Chillax!*" I shook my head. "Good grief, lady."

Slowly, she pivoted to my eyes. Once there, she articulated her displeasure in blades of ice.

"Miss Paige," I swallowed, realizing it was too late to retreat. "How about if we just let Freak tell us what he wants to do today? He's a big boy. He's been in the television business longer than any of us. He knows what's at stake." I licked my lips. "A few days ago, he fell from 20,000 feet and an exploding airplane. Him, not us." I gathered myself. "Freak gets to call the shots."

She launched a scowl that could sink a thousand ships. I glanced at Steve, needing any excuse to look away, trying to stay afloat as best I could.

Eventually, Saundra reached for her water bottle on the table corner of the couch. After two token sips, she excused herself to use the bathroom. We averted our eyes as she strode from the room, thankful that our little band of brothers could finally resume practicing the art of how to breathe.

"Guys," whispered Steve," that's really not her." He checked the bathroom door. "It takes a lot of pressure for Saundra to get that ugly. Outside pressure. From those much higher up."

"How often," I asked, "do you have to put up with this?"

"Too often, I'm afraid."

"A spiritual attachment," said Freak. "Another Dark Rider. *Ambition.*"

"Okay," she said, returning from the door to her seat. "What shall we do today?" She pulled out her stylus and opened her phone's note app.

"I want," said Freak, gently but firmly, "to be the one who decides when you can put me back on the news."

"Yes. You've said that. I agree."

"I need to hear from the Lord before I make my next move. It is critical today for me to listen to what God is trying to say."

"Meanwhile, the world spins... waiting."

"As you say, the world spins. With or without your next report."

She forced a smile. Nodded.

Silence settled, unsettling us all. I glanced at my watch. Way too early for a beer. Still, a chilled Dark Mama... a cold chocolate milk stout....

"Hey," I said, "I've got a swell idea. Let's blow this popsicle stand. Let's get out of here."

Wilcox stiffened.

"Where?" asked Freak.

"My place. The cabin. I need to retrieve my cell phone and find my wallet. And I should check on the locks. Plus, I could really use some fresh underwear."

Steve snickered. "Too much information, Bro."

"As you know," said Wilcox, "the Elkhead Lodge provides laundry and dry cleaning services as part of our package."

"You don't get it," I grinned. "I like variety. Ask Saundra. My accumulation of jockey intimates has become a vast collection."

Andy gave me an odd look. Saundra almost broke her frown.

"I like it," said Freak. "I'd like to see my tomb again. To thank the Lord... and to listen. To get a feel for the place where you dug me out. And to pay homage to the miracle tree that broke my fall... and signed my face."

My stomach lurched. Hmm.

"Freak," asked Saundra, "would it be permissible for Steve and I to come along?"

He studied her for a moment, then nodded yes.

"And may we bring our gear?"

"Yes," he sighed. He slowly gazed around the circle. "Does anyone have a Bible? I need to do a little reading today. It is imperative that I regain my focus before I return to the air."

"Mom keeps one at the cabin," I said. "She'll get a big kick out of knowing that the world-renowned Reverend Bill Jacobs used her Bible to check in with his Boss."

Steve put down his napkin. "We all need some fresh sky." He stood. "I'm game!"

"Agent Wilcox," asked Saundra, "what do you think?" She leaned forward onto the overstuffed pillow she'd pulled into her lap, then batted her lashes ridiculously, tapping her stylus to her lips. "Can you and your team pretty please put together a plan for us?" Somehow, she managed to excise every particle of sarcasm from her voice. "Might you also be able to provide escorts... and perhaps a contingency or two?"

I could hardly stifle my laugh.

"That's my job," he grinned.

18
THE RIDE

I pulled out my keys.

"Uh-uh," said Wilcox. "You won't be needing those."
He held the glass door as we filed out from the lodge into
the crisp mountain air. Two Summit County uniforms and
an indeterminate number of plainclothesmen restrained
the media packs, who bayed annoyingly, at least for now
beyond arm's reach.

"My teams will be providing all of the necessary
transportation," said Wilcox.

"What," I gloated, "is my red beastie too conspicuous?"
I spotted my SUV Ford, floating impressively above my
upgraded 20 inch custom chrome wheels. My hands and
right leg tingled, eager after too many days of restraint to
finally again experience a restoration of power.

"No... your red paint is not the problem." Wilcox nodded towards the street. "But today's ground plan does not include riding around in your car."

"Rig," I said, following his nod.

A hulking pair of modified military Command and Control Humvees rambled up the drive. It took me a moment to absorb what was happening. I'd never seen armored special op patrol versions of a Hummer in the valley before. They must have been sling-loaded in from Fort Carson on a couple of cargo choppers. They rolled past my beastie as indifferent as rhinos to a lady bug.

Hmm.

"So," I sighed. "I don't suppose I get to drive one of those?"

"Naw. Thanks for the offer, though." He grinned. "We've got the rigs and drivers already in place."

I sat up front with our special op driver, looking down on the world from the scout vehicle. I had positioned myself to audibly confirm for him the few turns we would need to negotiate in order to attain the cabin.

He indulged me, probably having already memorized every road in the valley on his flight over.

While rumbling out the drive and past my beastie, I realized my comparison of rhinos to a lady bug had not done my girl justice. More like two orcs strolling indifferently past a cute sleeping halfling. I tipped a nod toward my resting Hobbit, congratulating her for having learned her lessons. This time, she'd parked in a spot pointing at a neglected service road exit branching from the main drive.

If hostile journalists tried another ambush, she would slip through the side gate before they could cinch their noose.

They would not get away with blindsiding her twice.

Back onto the striped pavement, Wilcox reviewed strategies from the back seat. I split my attention between federal logic and the visceral rush of riding perched on such power, mounted securely behind the imposing armor plates of this leviathan. I longingly surveyed the bewildering array of instruments in the cab, and I covetously inventoried the arsenal of weaponry stowed around me only a reflexive hand snatch away.

"... organized demonstrations of strength are critical right now," droned Wilcox, enjoying the ride as much as me, but for reasons all his own. "The helicopters and uniformed military presence together convey a warning of attentiveness. We want to send a message."

"Message?" asked Freak. He shifted behind me, cocooned in his now-signature orange parka, appearing as mildly anxious as his scars would permit.

"If someone is out there," said Wilcox, "and I must emphasis the *if*, then we want them to know that the valley has been thoroughly locked down. The few roads in and out of Summit County this time of year are under tight surveillance. The enemy is going to need a better plan than just pointing a gun and pulling a trigger. We're telegraphing a loud message to any possible assassin: they will need to formulate a complicated extraction strategy. On top of everything else, their need to develop an escape plan is buying us more time."

"I see," I said, trying to imagine what it would feel like to crank that massive wrapped steering wheel with my greedy mitts. I tried to conjure the thrill of fussing with the glowing symphony of high-tech instrumentation. To picture myself pulling off on a logging road and gearing down to test the undercarriage clearance and stream-fording capacities of this Beast.

I spotted a set of winch controls, then had to sit on my hands to resist tugging on one of the glistening black tootsie-pop sticks.

"Sir," I addressed our driver, "when you cable onto a tree, which moves first? The Humvee... or the mountain?"

He laughed. "It depends upon the objective of the mission."

We passed the hospital in Frisco. The white media tent in the parking lot pulsed slowly in the gentle gusts of breath exchange between Lake Dillon's Frisco Bay below and the nearby peaks rising to the west.

Hopeful television crews continued to loiter about the makeshift studio compound, waiting for who-knows-what. But their ranks had thinned a bit since the departure of Freak. Those who remained turned in confused jerks as we clattered by. Several immediately began to scramble. The big Denver Channel 5 live unit was already in position to follow, idling expectantly at the edge of the parking lot.

Saundra must have called in the tip.

I transferred my attention to the glowing LED screens monitoring our Command vehicle's rear and flanks. Another military driver transported the rest of our lodge party, holding column formation immediately behind us. Next came one of Andy's men in a Summit County

Sheriff's cruiser. Completing our platoon were a dozen or so live television units from the now-permanent stakeout at our resort. As luck would have it, they happened to be going our way, out enjoying Colorado's invigorating recreational opportunities and exercising their constitutional rights.

The rattling of our passage created a stir along the main drag.

Rubberneckers gawked from every intersection. Tourists fumbled with cameras in gift shop doorways. Dogs barked. Late-sleepers dropped their toast in continental breakfast lobbies.

By the time we began accelerating onto the I-70 freeway ramp, additional broadcast reinforcements had rolled out from the hospital and several motels, and all were now dutifully falling into line with our increasingly newsworthy convoy. Several civilian vehicles were swept into the wake of our parade, including a Subaru Crosstrek, two off-road pickups, and a rusty blue Astro minivan with Oklahoma plates.

Saundra and Steve were undoubtedly fuming.

They had to be furious that at least one of their pair was not sitting in the head vehicle with Pastor Freak and Agent Wilcox, stylus or camera in hand, poised to capture any secret exchanges between church and state. Not to mention Saundra's likely paranoia about losing scoops to trailing troops.

We exited down off I-70 and surrendered several units to Silverthorne stoplights, but more than offset our losses by gains from the Outlet Mall. North of the main business district, we began our thundering descent along the Blue

River highway. We made good time until we were forced at the far north end of town to slow again, nearly to a halt, when a car unexpectedly pulled out in front of us from the Last Stop Liquors drive.

I took it as an omen.

Obedient to fate, I squinted, trying to see if the young blonde might be peddling her wares at the cash register inside. The door and windows of the store simply mirrored back a blank flash, revealing nothing I could use.

Across the parking lot at True Blue Bible, the controversial unsanctioned sign now leaned against a little white church bus at the back of the plowed pad. Its lettering still faced Highway 9, still directing sinners and saints alike as to where they should park for a timely escape.

"Freak," I said, "that chapel over there might be right up your alley. Maybe we should check it out this afternoon on our way back to the lodge."

"Maybe," he agreed. "I definitely need a place to pray."

"I couldn't help but notice," he added, "that there was a Dark Mama Beer poster in the liquor store window. It had a really pretty woman in a black dress. That's your brand, right?"

"My new favorite. How'd you know?"

"I overheard you complaining to Steve about how you couldn't get any at the lodge."

He tapped my shoulder. "Dark Mama Beer... that is."

I chuckled. A sense of humor. Who would have thought. A couple six packs were still chilling in the cabin fridge, but I couldn't argue against the opportunity for some live chilling with that gorgeous clerk again.

"Agent Wilcox," said Freak, "perhaps we can stop back there this afternoon. Me for the church. Mark for his pretty-lady beer."

"Sure," said Wilcox. "Impromptu stops can be effective... as long as we stay alert. If anyone is trying to keep tabs on us, a little spontaneity will help to keep them guessing."

Guessing indeed. I grinned. Our column probably now stretched half a mile. It's not like they wouldn't see us coming.

At the Rock Creek turnoff, the Summit County sergeant behind Andy's Humvee hit his flashers. I watched in the rear monitor as he parked his car sideways, creating a roadblock to restrain the media train, allowing us some privacy while we geared down and began our final steep ascent up the slippery, rutted, and narrowing Keller Mountain climb.

Too bad for J.B's Repair Service and Rescue Winch. The lawman's barricade had just robbed Johnny of a week's worth of towing.

CABIN FEVER

The cabin's drive and turnaround were freshly plowed.
Expanded. Scraped flat, dry.

"Your work?" I asked, leaning to eyeball Wilcox
through the mirror.

"Not me," he grinned. "One of my teams."

Hmm.

The thought of government agents with heavy iron
blades inviting themselves onto our remote property, the
grating and swiping away a generation's worth of ruts and
character, did not sit well. It was a personal violation. This
felt categorically different than Saundra and Steve walking
around the cabin to hike up my tracks through soft snow
to visit Freak's tree.

Yellow caution tape stretched taut between lodgepole
pines for a hundred yards to either side of the cabin.

Every twenty steps or so, a bright cardboard "No Trespassing" sign was stapled to one of the dark trunks.

"Your work?" I asked again, nodding down the yellow line as our driver jammed the safety brake and locked the rig's gargantuan wheels.

"No, that was your dad's contribution. To be honest, it was a good idea. I agreed with him the signs might help keep some of the gawkers from tromping through your yard. We don't have the manpower to stay 24-7 on everything at once."

"You've been talking to my dad?"

"Of course. And he gave us a key. Not that we needed one."

"Is he here now?" I yanked the door lever open, but made no attempt to step out.

"No. We only met briefly, when I first arrived. He didn't even spend the night."

"Was that his idea... or yours?" I swivelled in my seat to face Wilcox head on. "It's not like Dad to drive all the way up here and not do a little hanging out. Who came up with the plan for him to drive back to Denver?"

"I did. That was my idea. But he saw the wisdom." Wilcox opened his door and climbed down, then came around to my side of Humvee. He placed a hand on my partially opened armored door. Then leaned close. "Seriously, Mark. I'm worried you still don't get it."

"You've got to be joking." I shook my head in growing frustration. "You ran my dad out of his own mountain home. Who do you think you are?"

"Grow up, kid." He bent even closer. "Who do *you* think I am?" He dropped his hand from the door and leaned back. "In case you haven't heard, several thousand of your fellow citizens were brutally murdered this past week. America is at war. Watch the news."

"I *am* the news," I snapped.

"Wrong. You're nobody. That crazy preacher friend of yours who calls himself an End-Time Prophet... *he* is the news." He nodded to the back seat. "Him... and the terrorists. And the dozen or more nations behind the terrorists. We're talking about a richly financed, highly organized, subversive global army that is eager to do everything in their power to turn our planet's clock back to the Dark Ages."

"Nobody really wants war," I said. "I mean, the terrorists do, but they'll never get away with it. The rest of the world will...."

"Will *what*?"

I shrugged.

"Open your eyes. You're looking at the *'will what.'* The rest of the world will do exactly what I'm doing right now. While you goof off drinking yourself silly and making cheap passes at the pretty girls, we've got the assignment of doing everything we can to stabilize the situation and make sure nothing escalates any further. Lord help us all if it does."

"The Lord," said Freak, "is not putting on the brakes this time. Trust me. The escalations are coming." He leaned forward into our conversation, making himself unmistakably present. "The Lord's dispensation of grace is ending. Look at the world. Mercy hasn't worked. Now the Lord will turn to judgment to set things straight. The Holy Spirit's season of restraint—the time of His active participation in the containment and suppression of evil—is drawing to a close. The wickedness of men will become more clear, even as the disasters and horrors of war grow much worse."

Wilcox shook his head sideways.

"See," he spat, nodding again at Freak. "That's what I'm talking about. If we're not careful, your friend here is in a position to push our planet into World War Three."

"Come off it," I said. "You've been reading too many of your department's own press releases. There's no way...."

"Fine." He stepped away from my door.

"You've got one hour," he said. "Go ahead, wander around. Show off for the lady. Collect your things. Then we head back. It's not safe, kid. Even if you're too dense to know it."

"Hold on," I protested. "This is private land. You can leave whenever you want, but you can't tell me how long I can stay on my own property. Just because you got away with intimidating my father...."

"*Mark!*" barked Freak.

He reached over the seat and sank fingers into my shoulder. "Wilcox is right. I sense great danger here. An ominous danger is now growing throughout the entire valley. Dark Riders have begun to circle... and to descend."

It was all I could do to keep from knocking Freak's clamped hand all the way back to the cursed day I'd found him. I closed my eyes, took a deep breath, and respectfully brushed his hand from my person.

America at war? World War Three?

I pushed through my door, past Wilcox, and dropped to the driveway. I looked back into the rig, across my empty seat to our square-chinned chauffeur, who sat stoically, hands at rest upon the leather-wrapped steering wheel.

"What do you think?" I asked. "World War Three?"

"Just following orders, sir."

I stepped away and shut the beast. I absently withdrew my keys and glanced towards our cabin's front porch with its useless locks.

"Yo... Mark!" Steve shouted from beside the other all-terrain tactical monstrosity further down the drive. "Are you going to give us a tour, or not?" Black equipment bags and Saundra stood waiting on my federally scraped dirt drive.

A cloud of breathy fog puffed thinly around each of us in the 9,000 foot air.

My cell phone was blinking, plugged in, fully charged.

"Is that your work, too?" I redirected the agent's nose away from my shelved personal effects to the private cache of my communications sitting beside a notepad near the kitchen sink.

"I hope," I continued, "that you found what you wanted. Or are you going to say it was my dad who plugged my phone in to charge?"

"Kid, you've got to stop making everything about you and your dad. It doesn't matter. There it is. Check your messages. And let's find Freak your mother's Bible so he can finally stop twitching and relax."

"What? You don't know in which drawer my mother keeps her Bible? Are you getting lazy, or what?"

Wilcox frowned.

My phone rang. I grabbed it, didn't recognize the number, and shut it off. I scooped up my charger and found my wallet where I'd left it on the table before heading out to snowshoe the other day. Then I turned toward my bedroom to restuff my duffle bag with everything I'd brought up for spring break, plus whatever else that would fit from my dresser drawers.

"Nice place," whistled Steve. He was pulling out his camera and heading my way.

"Nice view," added Saundra, drifting to a window. "Mind if we get a few shots?"

"I suppose," I said. "But better clear it with Wilcox first."

Wilcox grinned, satisfied. Nodded yes.

I showed them around, inside and out. Steve filmed everything.

Saundra clarified that for every five minutes of B-roll footage on a story like this, as little as five seconds might survive the final edit. I noticed Steve was unusually creative in his camera angles, putting a knee on chairs, dropping to the floor, poking out from behind a corner now and then.

Creative to the degree that sometimes Freak ended up in a frame, usually when he was looking the other way.

Unaware.

Through the back windows, it was obvious that dozens of investigators had come and gone over the past few days. Perhaps a rogue journalist or two had even made the trek. A wide, deep hard-packed trail now ran up from the deck into the forest, where only days before the route had been a challenging task even on snowshoes.

Leading the tour through the back door, I noticed my liquor store empties and shards had been removed. As had the rest of my full bottles and the novel I'd left splayed on the glass deck table in the sun.

I lifted an eyebrow at Wilcox. He grinned, then tipped his head towards the refrigerator and bookshelf inside.

From the back deck, I pointed to where our property line ended at the aspens and small lodgepoles, and where the Eagles Nest Wilderness Area began.

When Saundra pressed for more, I briefly explained the legal and working relationships between grandfathered family properties like ours, and the occasionally-accommodating complex policies of the White River National Forest Administration.

My lecture was all rather droll, with gratuitous references to the federal government liberally salted throughout. I figured none of it would end up in the edited story anyway.

So I gave Saundra what she seemed to want.

THE CURSED TREE

"And here," said Sandra, professionally punching each word into her handheld mic, "behind me, is the trail descending from the deep snow and dark shadowed conifers of the White River National Forest."

my direction.

Steve rose smoothly from his squatting position on the deck until the camera angled down to where Saundra now pointed at the packed footprints near her feet.

"And it is here that—only four days ago—high school English teacher Mark Hanson dragged the seemingly lifeless body of Reverend Bill Jacobs from what would have otherwise have been his icy grave."

"Nice." Steve dropped the camera from his shoulder. "Even better the second time."

"What do you think?" she asked, glowing in my direction.

"I think you're amazing. Seriously. You come alive when the camera is rolling. You're really good at what you do."

She beamed. "Thanks. At times, it feels like I was made for reporting. My mother has an old video of me as a child pretending to interview our cat."

"Yes," agreed Freak, "you have a gift." He caught her eye and held it.

Freak concluded, carefully selecting his words. "Saundra, you were made for such a time as this."

It could have been the mountain air. She seemed to flush.

"Esther," she replied. "You're comparing me to Esther. Should I be flattered... or offended?"

"Oh, definitely flattered." Freak seemed sincere. Saundra appeared delighted.

"Esther who?" I asked. I occasionally taught a Bible as Literature class, so I knew the reference. But I was curious as to where their exchange might go.

"Esther nobody," interrupted Steve. "Look, the sun is going to be manageable for another twenty minutes at best. And Wilcox is over there arguing with Andy about whether we've even got time to hike up the trail as it is. We've got to get moving. Otherwise, we might as well skip shooting the tree and head back to town right now."

Saundra smiled again at Freak. "As agreed, we'll be very respectful with the edit." She nodded with profound encouragement and promise. "Nothing sensational. No sideshow effects." She waved her hand. "Please, for the sake of my job... let us record this."

Freak turned from her to me. "What do you think, Mark? We don't want Saundra to lose this assignment. But I'm still not hearing anything from the Lord. You call it. What do you say... *wingman*?"

Saundra swung my way, now nodding her accomplished encouragements and promises at me.

She'd never glowed more radiantly. That close. The angle of the sun and the dropping temperatures raised a whimsical glimmer to her cheeks.

"Steve's right," I enthused. "Let's get moving. Before it's too late."

With a packed trail, the going was relatively easy and the distance somewhat shorter than I remembered.

Steve kept filming the whole time, sometimes from ahead, sometimes behind. As far as I could tell, he was careful to avoid recording from Freak's left side. Saundra kept us all loose and talking. She stopped us several times to jot notes or to set up a retake on a particularly good question or interesting response.

Mom's Bible proved to be a compelling prop. Freak eagerly reached into the parka's enormous vest pocket to retrieve and wave the big black New King James whenever the occasion allowed.

He must have done Shakespeare in college. And maybe he was recapturing the rhythms of his television show. His timing was perfect, and he instinctively knew whenever the Good Word could use a little extra wind to drive home an especially salient point.

"Freak," she asked, "do you have any thoughts about those who attacked the planes? Standing here, near where you fell to earth, how do you answer their claims to have struck the West to bring glory to Allah... and to spread the truth of their holy religion?"

Freak hesitated. He closed his eyes, then reached into his vest. He opened the book to the prophet Isaiah.

"Woe to those who call *evil*... good," Freak bellowed. "And woe to those who call *good*... evil." He lowered the Bible.

"And woe to those who say such deceptions and distinctions do not matter. The Lord shall soon bring utter clarity to mankind... moral clarity that will bruise and burn."

He pointed to the heavens.

"Woe to those who murder the innocent, those who drop children and women from the sky. And woe to all of the twisted self-righteous sinners who greedily kill and exploit under the cover of the name of God."

He tucked the Bible back into his vest.

"Their Day of Straightening is at hand."

A few of America's military adventures and economic experiments came to mind, and I suddenly hoped Freak was woefully wrong.

Maybe a woe to *some* of the sinners... but not to all?

Between stops, Steve confirmed that he'd strapped on my Bear Paws the last time he'd been up this way. Evidence of his snowshoeing ineptitude littered the parallel trail, which was still punctuated with frequent fat snow angels and butt blotches.

In a spirit of full disclosure, Saundra then confessed she'd never made it up through the deep snow as far as Freak's tree. With Steve's help, she'd generated a voiceover from the Chanel 5 broadcast truck later at the hospital lot.

Then Freak surprised us all by admitting he was beginning to recall parts of the trail he'd forgotten that he'd seen. He paused, stopping us all in a distinctive stretch of the path, in the midst of an unusual hodgepodge of Englemann spruces, lodgepoles and blackjack pines.

"I remember...." Freak was beginning to pant in the thin altitude air. His scars flamed from the exertion and cold. "I remember finally being able to force an eye to flicker open somewhere around this spot."

He lifted his head to the soaring conifer heights.

"Every fiber of my body was in shock, paralyzed from the trauma of the impact. Mark was dragging me by the hood, pulling me by my parka. I remember fading in and out of this dreamlike experience. It was almost like floating on water, tubing along a riverbank... trees overhead, occasional patches of sky. The drop from the plane had been mind-blowing. Without reference points, without weight. Just burning, screaming air. And the angels."

He nodded.

"But here," he swept his hand up and down the trail, "this became more real than the fall. It was here that I knew for certain I was still alive."

"How so?" prodded Saundra, glancing to Steve to confirm he was rolling.

"The snow. As Mark pulled me along, my parka kept creeping up until it was higher than my belt. The snow starting slipping into my pants... and shorts."

We laughed. "I remember feeling the freezing slush as it worked its way down deep... way down. I remember thinking: 'Lord, thank you for providing soft snow to cushion my fall. But I'm safe now. Is there any chance you could turn up the heat?'"

We all laughed again.

"Why didn't you say something," I asked. "At that point, for all I knew, I was dragging a corpse."

"Are you kidding?" he snorted. "The way you were wheezing and floundering, I figured if you knew I could speak, then you probably would have tried to reverse the situation. You would have made *me* carry *you*."

I sensed we were drawing near before I spotted the landmark pine.

At once, all of us stopped dead in our tracks.

Saundra gulped. Steve adjusted his camera, unsteady.

Desecrated.

Me, Steve and the feds had not been the only ones to visit Freak's tree.

Some person—or persons—had turned Freak's saving tree into an unholy shrine.

Blood and entrails had been sprinkled and splashed everywhere. On the snow, against the trees, and even onto the last few steps of the trail. Tufts of feathers were tied with fur and animal skins and knotted into grotesque fetish totems that dangled from many of the lower branches of the once-stately pine.

The area where Freak crashed through branches and slid to rest was now all an open trench, presumably dug wide by the investigative teams.

But it hadn't been some forensics geek who'd done this. Who had doused the crater with urine and excrement down into the pit's base. And who had flung into the hole the eviscerated, crushed and mutilated bodies of several small pets.

I had guessed that Freak was a tongues-speaker from the first time I'd heard his mumbling. In the face of this, he erupted in loud, unnatural utterances from some place very deep. Deeper than I'd ever been. I tried to understand, torn between the horror of the shrine and my fascination with what flowed from his lips. But I couldn't make out a word of it. Saundra kept shaking her head, first at the defiled tree, then Freak, then looking away.

Steve caught it all.

Finally, Freak drew forth my mother's Bible and began selecting passages and reading at length, prophesying through tears at the curse and the symbol that had been carved upon his tree.

A deep, three-foot wide swath of bark had been hacked and peeled all the way around the pine, through the tender cambium layer of life, and into the heartwood core... condemning the tree to certain death.

There, on that naked, warped wooden slate, letters were crudely formed, sliced by some wicked blade. Words had been gouged deeply, above and below what appeared to be a savagely carved upside down cross.

And the whole corrupt business was smeared with blood.

From where Freak was preaching, Steve had no choice. In order to get both the prophet and the cursed tree in the same frame, the cameraman was forced to find a position to the pastor's left side.

If things had played differently, Steve might have won an award for that clip.

The shot opened with a tight frame on Freak's throbbing, flaming wounds... his lips pleading in tongues, his scars glistening in tears. The shot pulled back to capture his orange parka on a canvass of dark forest shadows and red-splattered snow. Then, it slowly panned and pushed in, past the black Bible in Freak's trembling hand, down tight to nothing but the tree's wretched rant, etched in blood:

FREAK
FROM
HELL

COME
HOME!

And, stretched there below the curse, was a blood-drenched voodoo doll. Primitive, spread eagle... long rusty spikes driven through its hands and feet.

It was crucified, nailed into the long, tangled forelock of a beast.

The bloody, freshly severed head of a white horse.

That was about the time when Freak stopped reading.

Stopped praying.

Stared.

Dropped my mother's Bible into the snow.

My gaze shot back and forth between the tree and Freak as our miracle boy slowly raised a shaking arm and pointed a quivering finger at a thick branch that swayed gently over the blasphemous pit.

"There," he gasped. "It's the Devil himself."

Saundra screamed.

In retrospect, I *might* have noticed a few inches of movement. I may have heard a soft, unearthly cackling.

But I don't think so.

For all I know, a raven had flown up from some dumpster in the valley to peck at one of the meat chunks suspended in the reticent air. News broadcasts by other stations later documented that an odious flock of the vile birds had laid claim to the site. The dark-winged watchers tormented reporters and rodent scavengers alike, whoever gathered to feast upon any scraps they could find.

The next day, when we all finally had the psychological margin to sanely debrief, Freak corrected himself. Even in his Twilight Zone version of reality, he came to doubt whether he had actually seen Satan himself mocking us from the tree. "A territorial spirit," he said. "An arch-demon at best."

Freak figured Lucifer would have farmed out the privilege of mocking us to some lesser spirit. The task would have gone to some other tormentor, perhaps one who was already attached to the cult and who had been on the assignment from the beginning.

Saundra, of course, was understandably livid for the next three days. "You did it again," she accused. "Why is it, Freak, that you keep doing this to me? First angels, now demons. Please, from now on... keep your crazy visions to yourself."

Still beneath the tree, though, there wasn't a whole lot of reflecting and introspecting going on.

Saundra kept screaming.

Freak scooped Mom's Bible from where it had fallen in the snow. He flipped open to a Revelation something-or-another passage and started reading again, now in a rather imposing big-pulpit voice. I squinted at the branch for all I was worth, then grabbed Saundra and rotated her into my chest. I held her as close as I could until the hysteria settled into quiet sobs.

Steve stuck to it with his camera, doing what he always loved to do best.

Eventually, Wilcox and one of the drivers arrived and pulled us from the scene.

They were forced to get a little rough with Freak in order to break the spell, for which they were later appropriately apologetic.

"We will stop at the chapel," consoled Wilcox, loading us back into the Humvees. "We'll make time for the church. We can try to find the pastor... maybe he will sit with Freak and talk this through. Hopefully, there will be somebody there to provide whatever it is Freak might need."

"*Prayers*," whispered Freak. "We all need prayers."

21
THE LITTLE CHURCH

Pastor Gilford wasn't at his church. Thankfully, though, the chaplain was right next door, aft of the chapel, peering through the curtains in the front room of the church's dowdy little parsonage.

"Freak, you might want to pull up your hood...." I nodded at the swelling mob behind the improvised crowd control line. "Unless you're ready to make this your official coming-out debut, you'll probably need to yank the drawstring tight again one more time."

He sat shaking behind me in the Humvee, at the window on the right. Any footage recorded so far was only catching his good side. Sheriff Andy and Agent Wilcox had telephoned back and forth with their teams continuously during our drive down from the cabin. A detective and a forensics team were immediately dispatched to the site to rope things off and sift for clues. Several additional law enforcement units were summoned to prepare for our arrival at the church.

Freak hesitated. He lifted his hood, then tugged it snug.

"I'll scope things out," I said, pushing out my door. "Then I'll wave you in... if I can."

"Okay," he murmured. "Thank you... *wingman.*"

"Wilcox," I asked, "are you in on this, or not?"

He frowned, then opened his door and dropped to the gravel, suddenly a quick step ahead of me.

It took us several rounds of knocking to coax Pastor Gilford to the parsonage door.

"Sorry," he complained. "I wasn't expecting anyone. What's going on with those army trucks and flashing lights and everything? Am I in some kind of trouble?"

"No," replied Wilcox. "Of course not. But we're hoping that you can help us with something...."

"I'm Mark Hanson," I interrupted, reaching for the pastor's boney hand.

Gilford appeared more gaunt and frail in his slippers than I could have imagined when seeing him in his boots and puffy jacket in front of his ill-fated church sign. I lightened my handshake for fear of breaking something within his fragile grip.

"Sir," I smiled, "we're finding ourselves caught up in some really nasty religious business, and we need a preacher."

"Okay." He quickly released my handshake, looked at Wilcox, then back inside. He opened the door another six inches. "I'm Pastor Rodney Gilford. How can I help you?"

"We're hoping," said Wilcox, "that you'd be willing to talk to someone. Maybe pray with him."

"Him?" He nodded toward the Humvees. "Did you bring him here... the man from the plane?"

"His name," I said, "is Reverend Bill Jacobs. He's pretty upset. Something happened."

"Yes. I know who he is. But I wasn't sure which name I should use...."

"Would you," asked Wilcox, "be willing to talk with Reverend Jacobs?"

"Of course," he conceded. "I would never turn away anyone who needed help." He nervously glanced past us to the cameras and the noisy throng in the parking lot.

"Wonderful," I said. "Should we bring Freak here... or over to the church?"

"Goodness," he gasped, shrinking back. "Not in my home." He called over his shoulder, "Honey...." A woman much larger than Gilford shuffled forward from the shadows.

"Sarah, would you please get me my jacket. And call Elder Bates. Tell David to meet me at the church. Right away."

The creaky pews were unpadded, but clean, as was everything else in the little sanctuary. Freak and I sat on the front bench, facing a modest oak podium on a small red carpeted platform. Pastor Gilford and the gray-whiskered Elder David Bates faced us, fidgeting from folding chairs they'd pulled from a side closet. Agent Wilcox leaned beside a window, arms folded, watchful. Saundra and Steve waited outside, frustrated, milling restlessly about like all of the other media teams forced to endure yet another Freak story blackout.

Gilford swallowed. He regathered himself, apparently fighting a spontaneous bout of stomach flu.

"I'm sorry," intoned the pastor. He dropped his gaze to Freak's hands, "but I'm really not sure what you want from me."

"I've told you everything," sighed Freak, his scars blazing. "I've just been placed under a blood curse. The curse needs to be broken by Christians who know how to pray. I need to be spiritually strengthened."

"Don't you have friends?" Gilford turned to me. "Doesn't he have some people on his staff... some clergy friends back in California or something?"

I started to respond, then realized I had no answer.

Freak stretched his hand. "Pastor Gilford," he pleaded. "*Pray* with me. Ask God to protect me, to show me what I need to do." He opened his hands. "Anoint me with oil. Whatever the Holy Spirit says."

"Oil?" Gilford shuddered. He rotated to the man beside him. "Elder Bates, you've been very quiet."

We all turned to Bates.

Bates looked a bit less the rube in his plaid hunting vest and duckbill cap than he had on Friday with a shovel and dirty bib overhauls. Other than a few egg-yolk dribble knots in his unkempt salt-and-pepper beard, he presented relatively mountain average.

He cleared his throat.

"Reverend Jacobs...." Bates focused on Freak's eyes. "We've all seen you on television before. Here in this church, we may not agree with you about everything you preach, but most of us believe you're right about the end of the world—about the rapture and the tribulation... and all of the other theoretical eschatological whatnot."

Freak smiled, faintly.

"Personally, I'm not sure what to make of you falling from the plane into our community. I'm almost speechless, seeing a big celebrity pastor like you sitting here in our little church during Holy Week. I just finished cleaning up the mess the kids made on Palm Sunday, and now you're in our pews, talking about a cult or someone splashing blood around and making animal sacrifices just up the hill. A big shot like you is asking *us*... for help. And with Easter only a few days out. It all feels almost kinda supernatural or something."

As his words sank in, I felt a bit unhinged myself.

It had been a lot of years since I'd been in a church, let alone since I'd considered observing a Holy Week. For me, Easter was an occasional bookend for spring break. The annual Chocolate-Bunny holiday had become no more extraordinary than any run-of-the-mill Groundhog Day. Yet, to hear this simple Bates fellow summarize the present week as a supernatural whatnot... it all gave me pause.

Bates glanced at his own pastor, then back to his guest's scars. He studied Freak's face, puzzling over the damage like a broken porch step that could go either way: perhaps to be repaired, or maybe requiring a full replacement.

"We don't use oil in this church," said the elder. "I guess here at True Blue Bible, we believe oil was only supposed to be used in olden times."

Bates shimmied his gaze from the scars over to Freak's eyes. "But I would be honored to lay hands on your shoulder and to pray for you." He glanced at Gilford. "We did a laying on of hands once when we prayed for Henrietta's chronic carpal tunnels, right?"

"Didn't work, though," reminded the pastor.

Bates absently tugged his beard. "Probably didn't hurt, though, huh? The dear saint seemed to appreciate the effort all the same." He shifted his gaze to me. "She's dead now, of course. Not from the carpals. It was a bad run of heart issues that liberated Henrietta from this old sad trail of tears."

Pastor Gilford squirmed, resigned. He rose from his chair and mounted the single step of the low stage. Behind him, ten feet past the lectern, a stark wooden cross hung on the white plaster wall. To the left was an empty, aqua-colored baptismal tank. He returned from the pulpit with a worn leather Bible.

"The Word of the Lord," he reassured himself, patting it with his right hand. He hesitated. "Reverend Jacobs, what would you like us to pray for?"

Freak shook his head. "Anything. Everything." He implored with his hands. "Pray however the Lord leads you. As I said, I sense a heavy spirit of witchcraft and demonic oppression. I've been cursed through some kind of pagan occult ritual. I need supernatural protection against satanic assignments that have been declared against me when animals were killed...."

Gilford held up his slightly gnarled hand, agitated.

"Yes, yes," he said. "We've heard all of that." He shifted, squaring himself, folding his hands on his closed Bible, glancing around the circle. "I am certain that out there in your left-coast mega church—and on your big fancy television show—thousands of people probably take curses and chanting and such nonsense seriously. But this is the real world. Around here, we're not all fancy and complicated. We're just simple, practical mountain folks. We knock the heads off chickens and butcher livestock for our meat lockers every week. A dead animal and some empty words are nothing to fear. As I said, around here, we're not intimidated by a little phony mumbo-jumbo. We're not into superstition."

"*Somebody* is into it," observed Freak. "Throats were slit and animals were ritually sacrificed—and not for supper—only a few miles from your front door."

"Probably some kids from Denver," said Gilford, looking exasperated. "Probably some teenagers who drove up to the mountains on a joyride with too many horror movies in their heads. City kids today have way too much time on their hands."

Freak started to protest, then adjusted his focus, past Gilford to gaze upon the cross. "Lord, have mercy," he sighed.

"Uh... Pastor...." The elder appeared troubled.

"Yes, Bates."

"You said a minute ago that we are all just practical mountain folks."

"And?"

"Do they have mountains in Florida?"

Gilford turned to me. "Bates is alluding to the fact I used to live in Florida."

He turned back to his elder. "But now I live here in Silverthorne, so I speak on behalf of this entire mountain community."

"Oh."

Hmm. "I'm a native," I volunteered. "I've got history in this community."

"No kidding?" said Bates.

"I've been skiing up here in Summit County ever since I was knee-high to a marmot."

"Yes," Gilford shrugged. "And how do you feel about the magic oils and all of those other such superstitions?"

"I've got a cabin," I added. "It's up Bootlegger way. It's been in our family for three generations."

"Yes. Well. Then I suppose you know what I'm talking about...."

"In my experience," I grinned, "mountain folks kinda like to speak for themselves. And they don't usually eat their horses."

"Uh... pastor...."

"What is it now, Bates?"

"I'm from Green Bay. That's in Wisconsin."

"I know where Green Bay is."

"Hills. Some big hills. But no mountains. Lots of stubborn, independent-minded Germans. We're born to argue... and to speak for ourselves, so I kinda agree with Mr. Mark that...."

Gilford patted his Bible again, harder than before. He twisted towards Freak.

"My sister," said Gilford, "she lives in San Francisco. She tells me, Mr. Jacobs, that she's been to your church. She says it gets pretty wild. Things at your church are done Hollywood style. Not exactly decently and in good order."

"I'm sorry," sighed Freak. "I apologize for the inconvenience of all of this." Freak swallowed. "I'm feeling really badly about all of this hullabaloo. But I'd still like to pray. I desperately need to meet up with the Lord someplace where it is safe. Where folks worship God. A place where God likes to show himself. Are you still willing to pray for me?"

"Of course we can pray." Gilford opened his Bible near the middle, then randomly dropped his palm on a page. He stretched his fingers, at last ready to oblige. "We can always beseech the Lord, no matter what." He closed his eyes, sucked a big breath, and prepared to begin.

"My hand," he said, "has fallen to Psalm 19. I always like to start my holy intercessions with a few words of praise and thanksgiving." He glanced around the circle. "Let us pray. 'The heavens declare the glory of God, and the heavens display his handiwork. Day unto day utters speech, and night unto night reveals knowledge....'"

"Wait," I said.

Everyone opened their eyes in my direction. Gilford was clearly annoyed.

"Freak...." I ventured. "If they promise not to film anything, would it by okay for me to bring Steve and Saundra in for this? Both of them are pretty rattled right now. Maybe this would help them, like it might help you."

I lifted a hand. "After all, you spooked her pretty badly. You've got Saundra thinking she met the Devil."

Freak studied me, curiously. He closed his eyes for a moment, then nodded yes.

I looked at Gilford, who officially sealed the plan with a reluctant nod.

22 PRAYERS

Outside, it was a madhouse behind the media containment line. Photographers held cameras over their heads or dropped a knee, desperately seeking the perfect angle of me exiting the church, hoping to discover Freak somehow trailing in my wake.

I spotted Saundra.

Then Steve.

They were at the front of the crowd, frantically flip-flopping their attention between my exit from the church and a couple of reinforcements from their station news team who had driven over in their mobile broadcasting van. The Channel 5 mast was already partially raised for live remote uplinking.

Sheriff Andy met me halfway. He instructed me where to wait while he culled the crowd. Moments later, he returned with the Channel 5 elect.

"Mark, what's going on?" Saundra's stylus was already poised on a blank screen, bouncing only slightly with each brisk step. She had obviously taken notes on the fly many times before.

"We're off the record," I said. "This is personal. This is not for Channel 5. Nor for anyone else."

I reached for the chapel door handle. "Freak said I could bring you both in for prayer."

I whisked them inside and walked them down the center aisle to the front pew. Brief introductions were made. Steve carefully placed his camera on the floor and gently pushed it out of the way. Saundra grew uncharacteristically subdued. She studied the wooden cross, trembling slightly. She glanced at the twitching, wiry Pastor Gilford, then turned to Freak.

"Thanks," she said, meeting Freak's eyes.

"It was his idea," said Freak, tilting slightly in my direction. "But I agreed. Something wicked was unleashed at that tree." He leaned, softly adding, "You'll need all of the faith and protection you can get. Pray. Listen. And focus on the cross."

Steve glanced to the front of the church. "I'm not sure what I believe," he said, shaking his head. "I've never had a lot of faith."

"Leverage," encouraged Freak. "Bring whatever you've got. Even a mustard seed is plenty enough." He looked at me. "You, too, Mark. The cross. And whatever faith you can muster."

I shrugged.

"An hour ago," said Freak, directing his attention towards Saundra, "you saw the blood. This is not just a news story. This is life and death. Mine. Yours. Millions. We need to hear from God. Now."

"Is everyone here, now?" demanded Gilford, repositioning his fluttering hands upon his Bible. He briefly surveyed each of us, counterclockwise, in turn.

Meeting no objection, he resumed.

"Father God," he began to pray, "we have gathered here today, in your holy presence, to beseech you on behalf of your humble servants...."

After a few lines, I noticed Saundra had put away her phone. Wilcox had slid onto a bench. His head rested upon his hands, on the back of the pew in front of him. Even Steve's eyes were closed. Freak's lips had begun their silent quivers.

"... and in your mercy, O Lord, you have seen fit to bring us here as your flock, gathering us into this sacred assembly." Gilford was settling in now, finally finding the song in it all. "We are but simple sinners, yet you have loved us from your throne...."

I soon lost track of everything except the practiced music of his voice and the beauty of seeing Saundra vulnerable like that again. Breathing deep, eyes closed, somehow innocent, trusting, reaching....

"... and by the blood of your son Jesus Christ...."

Freak erupted in a wail.

His hands shot straight to the heavens. Tears began streaming down his scar. It might have been the mention of blood and Jesus. But there he was again, doing that glossolalia thing or whatever it was. His words made no sense, but the sounds he groaned were filled with passion. His body moved in waves and tremors. I had never seen a man who could get so wildly emotional so quickly.

It took me a minute to realize that Gilford had stopped praying. Instead, he was staring at Freak. Apparently in disgust.

"Stop that," he glared. Then, louder, "Stop it!"

Freak trailed off. He peered up through wet eyes, confused.

"We'll have none of that in my church," rebuked Gilford.

"None of what....?" Freak appeared dazed.

"Demon tongues!"

Freak recoiled.

Elder Bates stiffened. Steve shook his head.

Freak took a deep breath. "Pastor Gilford," he apologized, "sometimes when I pray, the Holy Spirit...."

"Hush." Gilford abruptly stood, then sat. He sized up his congregation of ignorant outsiders. "The Bible is *very* clear about this." He turned to me. "Are you able to interpret... do you know the meaning of these utterances?"

I shrugged.

He turned to Saundra, then Steve. "Are either of you able to interpret these unnatural incantations? Because, if not, then scripture forbids this to continue."

Saundra hesitated.

"San Francisco," she said at last. "I think I heard him praying for San Francisco."

The silence became awful. Freak sat stunned. Elder Bates twitched.

"Pastor," said Elder Bates, finally breaking the quiet with a whisper. "Pastor, I think that given the circumstances...."

"Circumstances?" Gilford thumped his Bible to the floor beside his chair. "Yes! Let's review the circumstances." He stood and began to pace.

His head bobbed and his gaze began darting back and forth in a sickening game of eye-tag with Freak's flaming scars.

"This man," he said, "falls from an exploding plane. But by some supernatural intervention, he lives. Everybody dies... but *him*."

For the second time, Saundra began to speak. "Pastor Gilford...."

"Then, this man walks into our church... admitting that demons surround him. Perhaps bringing his wicked, clinging devils into this very temple of God."

Saundra tried again. "Pastor Gilford, he prayed for God to have mercy on the people of San Francisco...."

"And then, at the mere mention of Jesus, he is thrown into a fit of mouth-foaming incoherence. He defies holy scripture by speaking gibberish at the very altar of God's sanctuary... by blaspheming in unnatural tongues."

"When God heals," declared Gilford, addressing everyone but Freak, "God creates beauty." He scooped up his Bible. "Yet this man's unregenerate face is a frightful obscenity." He paused, then continued. "Look at him." He pointed his Bible.

"This man's face is not just scarred. It is sealed... it is emblazoned with death and destruction. It has been marked with a claw."

I rechecked Freak's cheek. It certainly did look as if a paw might have taken a swipe or two. I felt sick.

"This man's face glows..." declared Gilford, "unholy... with the mark of a beast."

Freak winced. Then shook.

"We need to ask," concluded Gilford, "if this self-proclaimed Freak is a man of God... or an agent of the Devil? Is he here to bless us, or to...."

"Stop it!" gasped Bates, leaping to his feet.

"Pastor," he said, his voice filled with emotion. "You should be ashamed of yourself. This poor man has already been cursed enough for one day."

Gilford, stunned, watched Bates stride to beside Freak and place a hand upon his shoulder.

"I'm very sorry, Reverend Jacobs. All of you... I apologize for our pastor. He has been going through a lot these past few months."

He looked at Freak.

"We have all been under a lot of stress. This has been a rough year for our little church." He glared at his pastor. "But there is no excuse for this, Pastor. These people have sought prayer and solace within God's sanctuary, and you have heaped burning coals upon their distress."

"Elder Bates," protested Gilford, "look at his face. God would not have left him like that if this man was to be a true prophet for the glorious return of Christ...."

"Be still," urged Bates, "Pastor, I fear you will bring judgment upon yourself."

Freak held up his hand.

Somehow, he suddenly brought to a halt everything in the room but our breathing. He quietly studied Gilford. A pained tremor swept his brow.

Freak slowly stood. He turned to Gilford, then addressed him, using a tone that I'd never heard before. Speaking as if no one else was in the church but the two pastors... and God.

"Rodney," he said, softly shaking his head. "I'm so sorry about your cancer."

Gilford stuttered. "What... I don't...."

"Lord have mercy," said Freak. "I know this has been an ordeal."

"How...?"

"You have prayed. Many have prayed."

Gilford's face dropped. He glanced at Bates, but Freak's eyes never moved.

"Pastor Gilford," said Freak, his voice growing large and strong. "The Lord has heard those prayers. The tumor in your..." he paused. "The six growths in your colon. They are of the enemy. Would you like to be delivered... would you like to be healed... today?"

Gilford recoiled as if struck.

"You have an appointment with your oncologist tomorrow, don't you, Pastor Gilford?"

Gilford stopped breathing.

"The Great Physician," said Freak, his voice assuming an unnerving combination of presumed power and affected reverence, "our Lord and Savior Jesus Christ... the Holy Spirit has anointed me to bring glory to His mighty name. To set the captives free."

Freak stepped closer.

"The Holy Spirit is here—my hand grows hot, electric—to release you in this hour...."

"Stay back!" Gilford nearly knocked over his chair.

Freak stopped.

He suddenly again became aware of the rest of us. He turned back to Gilford.

"All you need to do is receive this, Rodney. This healing is yours. Give praise to the Lord, and allow me to place my hand over your stomach and let me pray...."

"I will NOT!" Gilford nearly screamed.

Freak jumped. His right hand, which had begun to extend toward Gilford, dropped and clutched over his own abdomen. Freak doubled low, staggered and almost fell to the church floor.

Bates caught the falling Freak by the arm, steadied him, then eased him back into his seat. The rest of us sat frozen, stunned.

Gilford squeezed his eyes. He opened them and dropped his head into his hands.

Finally, Gilford lifted his gaze to Freak.

"You had no right," he whispered. "Our heavenly Father is a gentleman. He is not a gunslinger." His voice gained feeble steam. "Circus tricks are for gypsies and the gullible masses, for those desperate superstitious cult followers who pay their dollar and...."

"Please," said Freak. "Forgive me." His eyes moved around our circle, pausing on me. "I do not play theater... not always." He finished his sweep, resting on Gilford.

"Again," sighed Freak, addressing the pastor, "I apologize. I will leave you in peace."

Freak rose and stepped towards the door.

"No," said Bates, yet again gently guiding Freak back into his chair. "I promised to pray with you."

He turned to Gilford.

"Pastor, you need to step away. I'm going to pray with these people." Bates eased Freak into a posture of submission, replacing his hand again upon Freak's shoulder.

Bates began to pray before anyone could stop him.

I watched as Gilford stiffened, scowled, then retreated from the circle.

After several minutes, they were softly praying in turns, Bates, Freak and Saundra. Freak especially began getting after it. Steve and Wilcox said nothing, but they stayed in the circle, attentive. Occasionally, a head would lift. Eyes would move to the cross, then eventually lower again into the dark quietude of closed lashes.

When I left, slipping out to get my beer, Pastor Gilford was still sulking.

As I softly closed the door, I saw him raise his cell phone and begin to record the scene.

He had positioned himself deliberately, to film from Freak's left side.

To catch the scars.

23
THE LIQUOR STORE

Sheriff Andy met me as I stepped out the chapel door.

"They're still praying," I said.

"How long?"

"Probably a while. They're on a roll. Wanna help me fetch some beer?"

"I'll escort you over," he grinned. "But I'm not going inside." He gestured toward the hungry photographers. "There's no way I'm going to let them catch me schlepping booze out while in uniform."

Andy marched me as far as the Last Stop Liquors entrance. At the door, he pivoted and settled into a parade rest, seams crisp, brows furrowed.

"Keep an eye on things," I chided. "Heads up...." I pointed to the biggest camera. "Do you see that zoom lens over there? If I'm not mistaken, that is actually a Soviet-made miniaturized bazooka. Give 'em hell, Andy."

She watched as I entered beneath the tinkling silver bell. She was waiting behind the counter, glowing smugly from her stool.

"Anything new?" I asked, heading directly her way.

She dropped from her perch. Then she unexpectedly bounded from around the back of the counter and circled over to my side of the till.

"I saw you drive by this morning," she said, stepping very close. "I couldn't believe it when you slowed down... but then you kept going."

"Just out for a drive," I joked. "Me and my three hundred best friends."

"Is that preacher man here with you right now? Is he hiding inside one of those army tanks?"

"They're not really tanks," I laughed. "They're Humvees. High Mobility Multipurpose Wheeled Vehicles."

"Oh," she grinned. "My bad."

A blonde ponytail swayed through the back of her embroidered trucker's cap, but it was her black T-shirt tucked into those tight jeans that held my eye.

"Silverthorne Colorado" was silkscreened in large white letters across the top.

Below the name was a cartoon image of a yogi. The monk figure was suspended in an orange hoodie, legs crossed, hands folded, elbows on knees. He was flanked by two chubby little cherubs, each extending pine branches toward the center. Their four evergreen boughs together formed an X, an implied landing spot directly below the hooded man's rump.

Beneath the X, stenciled in bold letters, were the words: "Ground Zero."

"Clever," I nodded. "Looks like your Frisco Kid has been pretty busy."

"He has. But so have you!"

"Nothing special," I said. "Nightly news. Saving the world. That sort of thing."

"I've been watching you," she smiled, "and I've been reading about you every day. I've lived here all my life, and this is the biggest thing that's ever happened in Summit County. Maybe in the whole world."

She laughed, then suddenly threw herself upon me with a wiggling hug.

"It's good to see you again," she beamed. "I was hoping you'd come in."

I was surprised by her warmth. Surprised... and delighted.

Although the store was unusually busy, activity was rapidly slowing and swinging in my direction.

"Good to see you, too," I said, stepping back. "I like your shirt."

"Everything is going crazy," she said. She drifted back around the counter and hoisted herself back onto her stool. "You've been amazing." She leaned forward. "And you've been great for the town. Great for business." She flipped a hand towards a Silverthorne Ground Zero shirt rack island a few steps to her right.

Judging by the empty slots, they were already sold out in several sizes.

"Your boyfriend's work, right?"

"My idea. His talent." She looked down at the design she wore and tugged on the stretchy fabric. "He's been working day and night. He's printing two new versions even as we speak. I think his 'Freak Fell Here' shirt is going to sell the best. We hope to really cash in on this. Maybe the golden ticket has finally turned up after all."

"How much do they cost?" I asked, moving to the rack of shelves. "I could use one of these. My pink 'Race for the Cure' pullover is starting to fade."

"For you," she laughed. "The first one is free." She paused. "Now that I think about it, take several. It'll be good advertising. After all, when it comes to Ground Zero, Mark Hanson marks the spot. You practically own Ground Zero... the actual site where he crashed!"

"Well, technically, he landed in the national forest."

"But you saw his miracle landing. You dug him out of your backyard. You saved the prophet."

"Sounds like another shirt slogan," I laughed.

"Huh?"

"Save the Prophet."

"Well, maybe...." she squinted toward the ceiling.

"If you decide to print them," I said, "put me down for a dozen. I kinda feel sorry for the guy some of the time."

"I'll let you know if we do." She smiled. "Meanwhile, help yourself to whatever we've got. Just make sure the cameras catch you wearing one from time to time."

I extracted an extra-large Ground Zero from the bottom shelf.

As I straightened, I noticed a different display. It was over against the wall, directly below the brewery advertising poster I had admired during my most recent visit a few days before. Back when the world made sense, when I was an unknown English teacher goofing off on a snowy spring break.

The poster remained as I remembered, except now it sported a huge price sticker. Beneath the provocative Dillon Beach Brewing towel scene, there now sat a tall box half-filled with tightly rolled posters. Adjoined to the poster carton was a wide shelf unit stocked with huge towels.

"Congratulations," I said. "It appears our Silverthorne poster girl has gone big time."

"Out of the closet," she laughed. "My boss finally admitted he knew it was me all along. He was just too embarrassed to say anything."

"A blusher, eh?"

"And married. Anyway, he says from now on, we can sell all of the merchandise we want. He just wants a fifty-fifty split."

"You move fast," I said, sauntering toward the wall. "How'd you pull all of this together so quickly?"

"My boyfriend already had the poster and the towel marketing projects in the works. Plus several other promotions we'll be launching next week. We only needed one lucky break." She smiled. "Thank you, by the way."

"My pleasure." I withdrew a towel and checked the tag.

"He has been working with one of the biggest printing shops in Denver. They've offered him a job as soon as things slow down up here. They really love his stuff."

I reached for a rolled poster. "I'll bet they *do* love his stuff," I grinned. "No doubt."

She gave me a puzzled look, then giggled.

"Hey," she squealed, springing from her stool. "I've got an idea."

She bounced to my side, then conjured a cell phone and snatched my towel before I could protest.

"A selfie!" she whooped.

I suddenly found myself in a flurry of T-shirt and swirling cotton fabric. Wrapped in her arms. Again delighted, again surprised. Her camera flew around us at arm's length, flashing high and low, snapping a quick succession of pictures culminating in one grand finale, a shot to capture the ecstasy of her warm wet lips upon my reddening cheek.

Customers had stopped shopping. Several now stood facing me, mouths gaping, Zinfandels and gin bottles drooping in my direction.

"Thanks," she tittered, unfurling from the towel and squeezing her phone back into her jeans.

Movement down the aisle caught my eye. I glanced over as a guilty-looking older man slipped an iPhone back into his sagging pocket.

I shook my head, savoring a bit of guilt myself, then followed her back to the register.

"The real reason I'm here," I said, making a small pile of the tube, the shirt and the towel, "is for another round of those Dark Mamas." I pushed my souvenirs in her direction. "Your long-necks were every bit as good as you promised. Now I want to share some with my friends."

"Friends... like Freak?" She slipped the shirt and towel into a brown paper bag. "Are you really friends with that crazy preacher man?" She folded down the top of the bag. "He fascinates me. And he scares me. I think he scares a lot of people. What's he like?"

Hmm.

"I don't think he's crazy," I said. "But he's certainly unique. There's something weird about him. It's hard to tell if it is authentic, or show. Probably a mix of both. Would you like to meet him?"

She paused.

"Not today," I added quickly. "But some other time. Freak has had a very rough morning. Right now, he's next door... praying in the chapel."

"Oh." She pushed the bag in my direction.

"Some people hate the pastor," I said. "The security guy staying with us says there are people who even want Freak dead."

"Wow."

"That's why," I added, "the government is providing protection. They've got us staying in an executive townhouse in a big fancy lodge up in Breck."

"So I've heard. And how are your other friends doing?" She rolled a rubber band down the poster tube, sliding it to the center. "They say Saundra Paige is staying with you. Along with some other people."

"She's fine," I said. "They're all okay."

"Saundra is very pretty. And very smart. Is the government making her stay with you?"

"No. I invited her. She said yes. It's been working out okay."

"She came by here, you know. I'll bet you're having quite an adventure... shacking up with a classy lady like that? Running around with a celebrity and everything."

"I guess."

I wasn't sure whether to shake my head or to clarify the situation.

"What about the beer?" I asked. "I'd like a couple more sixes of those Dark Mamas."

"Sorry," she said, nodding to the cooler. "Sold out. We've still got most of the others, though."

"Sold out?"

"I warned you. That's the problem with a great craft beer... by the time it catches on, it's all gone. The guys are working on another batch, but it won't be ready to bottle for a few more weeks."

"Hey," I said, waving up at myself on the security monitor overhead. "I see you're still filming your reality show."

By the time she looked up, the image had cycled from the two of us at the cash register to an outside view. The parking lot was even busier than before, teaming with more station trucks, police officers, cameramen and milling reporters.

Beside the security monitor above, the little television was streaming an afternoon news program.

"Of course," she joked. "Now that you've joined the regular action here, the networks are talking about extending our contract for another season. But they want you to sign an agreement that you'll appear in at least four more episodes."

I wandered back to the Dillon Beach cooler racks.

"I'm really glad," she said, "that you took the time to see me. Who could have guessed you'd become so famous in less than a week."

"You, too," I said, tossing a light salute in the direction of her sexy posters. I selected a six-pack and brought it to the register.

"I thought," she said, "that I might see you someday in the funny pages." She reached under the counter and came back up with a small stack of newspapers. "But I never expected to read about you on the front page."

"Here," she said, sliding the top paper across to me. "I don't know if you've gotten to this one yet... it just came out."

The Summit County News showed me in a small inset photo, grinning during my interview at the hospital. I was directing a finger towards the sky beneath the banner headline: "Local man witnesses Freak Fall Miracle."

The main front page photo featured a fuzzy, ridiculously enlarged picture that had been shot through the windshield of my red beastie. The image had apparently been snapped from the fallen porta-potty barricade that had cut off our hospital escape. Saundra was cropped out of the frame, but there I was again, on the right edge, glaring. My raised hand was closed in a fist, and I was angrily mouthing something. It might have been the name of the passenger in my back seat.

Freak's orange hood was pulled, and he was slumping. But his head was turned just enough to reveal part of his scar, vaguely discernible in the flash. The caption explained: "Renowned California televangelist Reverend

Bill Jacobs transformed by Fall into self-proclaimed Freak."

"Nice," I said, folding the paper and sliding it back. "Anything else of interest? I've been watching the news, but I've only been reading articles from the national newspaper they slip under our door at the lodge. The night raids and drone strikes in Iran, and those sorts of stories."

"Seriously?" she asked. She shuffled through the stack and pulled out another. "Here. You're going to love this one. It's as local as it gets."

The photo was a freeze-frame from Saundra's first interview. She was smiling, and Freak was shown in his facial mummy-wrap, reaching to pat her knee.

"Defying Death," read the headline, "with Message of Doom." The caption below expounded: "San Francisco pastor Bill Jacobs survived the Falling Skies slaughter only to declare himself God's Prophet for the Apocalypse."

I put my finger on the caption and looked up.

"He didn't exactly say that," I said.

"Keep reading," she nodded.

I skimmed the article until I came to my name, then stopped, stunned.

> Colorado resident Mark Hanson collaborates on the unlikely story, claiming he dug the prophet from a snowbank after seeing the plane explode. The pastor allegedly crashed in a tree near Hanson's Silverthorne mountain home.

> Calling the event a 'miracle,' Hanson has begun assisting and advocating for the End Times preacher. Against medical advice, Hanson

conspired to secretly whisk Jacobs away from the Frisco Trauma Center and into seclusion. Through the help of an alert journalist, the plot was thwarted. Authorities are now keeping the frequently-volatile duo under close surveillance.

More volatile than ever, I closed the paper and returned it to the pile.

"I think it's all pretty cool," she grinned. "Except maybe for the religious parts."

RANDOM QUOTES

I paid in cash. As I gathered my purchases from the counter and waited for change, I followed her puzzled gaze to the screens above.

"Look," she pointed.

The security monitor captured the two of us at the counter, slack-jawed, staring at the ceiling.

But on the television screen next to the monitor, there I was again... beside myself, on a news feed. I was shown exiting a white church and walking with Sheriff Andy across a gravel parking lot to a liquor store entrance.

"Turn it up!"

"... only minutes before," panted the male voiceover, "when the Reverend Bill Jacobs arrived from the crash site in a military Command Humvee and entered the church." The shot switched to a slow pan of the armored lead vehicle, the church, and then the crowd control line. The camera finally settled on a familiar Channel 5 News reporter wearing a heavy jacket, standing with a hand-held mic.

"Beside me," said the journalist, "we have Pastor Rodney Gilford, leader of the church."

I spun around and peered between the signs and decals of the Last Stop Liquor's huge storefront window. There, at the back of the lot, Gilford stood in the midst of an impromptu press conference, waving his Bible and entertaining questions from Channel 5's live reporter, Tom Jackson.

I swung my attention back up to the television.

"Yes," insisted Gilford, "Mr. Jacobs is still inside."

Pastor Gilford fidgeted in front of his "Escape Forever" billboard, which leaned against the white bus in such a way so the block lettering of "Bible Church" could still be read.

"He came into our church, uninvited." Gilford turned from Tom Jackson to one of the other microphones thrusting in his direction. "The man demanded we sprinkle him with oil. When I refused, he became upset. And when I prayed the name Jesus over him, he flew into a rage and began babbling in demon tongues."

"Do you know," asked Tom Jackson, "what it was Reverend Jacobs might have been saying?"

Gilford hesitated. "His face is monstrous."

"Did he say anything you can recall?"

Gilford shuddered. "You have no idea how hard it is to look at him. It's as if Satan himself raked the man's cheek with a set of demonic claws."

Jackson stepped closer. "And what did Reverend Jacobs say? Did this self-proclaimed prophet of the Apocalypse make any predictions that you could understand?"

"I'm not saying that Jacobs *is* the Devil," said Gilford. "But there is definitely something supernatural going on... that is for sure. In my opinion, he has been marked by the Beast." He shrugged. "What else could it be?"

"But what did he *say?*" insisted Jackson. "Surely he said something you could understand?"

Gilford reached for Jackson's mic, then dropped his hand and leaned forward instead.

"He named California," said Gilford. "He pronounced a curse on the people of San Francisco." Gilford licked his lips, glancing from reporter to reporter. "Jacobs wants the city of San Francisco to be destroyed... because of all of the homosexuals."

The next thing I knew, I was pushing my way through the crowd.

"Lies!" I shouted. "What a bunch of BS!"

Tom Jackson was the last reporter to clear from my lane.

Suddenly, I stood confronting Gilford, face-to-face.

Cameras rolling.

"You jerk," I spat. "How can you stand there with a Bible and lie like that?"

He cowered, sputtering.

"Inside the church," I said, turning to the cameras, "Pastor Gilford claimed he couldn't understand a single word of what Reverend Jacobs was praying. Now he is saying that Freak made predictions about San Francisco."

I wheeled back to Gilford. "When were you lying? Then... or now?"

His eyes grew wide.

"I was there," I continued. "The only person who said anything about San Francisco was Saundra Paige... from Channel 5 News."

The mention of her hallowed name evoked a chorus of murmurs.

"Saundra was praying with Reverend Jacobs... and Saundra said she heard Freak praying *for* the city. Not against it." I glared at Gilford. "Freak wasn't cursing the people of San Francisco, he was crying out to God, begging for God to show them mercy. And I can testify... Freak said absolutely *nothing* about the gay community."

"Could you understand him?" asked Gilford, gaining courage. "How do you know he didn't pray judgment against the sinners?"

"Mark Hanson," interrupted Jackson, pressing the mic close to my chin. "You are the high school teacher who rescued Reverend Jacobs... you're the man who dug him from the deep snow. Have you heard him making any other End Time predictions in the past few days?"

"No," I said, struggling to compose myself. "All I can tell you is that he is inside the church, right now... praying. Trying to listen. He tried to pray for Pastor Gilford; he prayed that God would heal this man. But

Gilford drove him away. Reverend Jacobs weeps when he prays. I have never met anyone who works so hard to hear from God."

Another reporter attempted a question, but Tom Jackson shifted a shoulder and plunged his mic back into my face.

"Mr. Hanson, you have been with Jacobs almost day and night ever since the first hour of the disaster. How do you explain his survival... and his face?"

"I have no explanation," I said. "And I make no apologies. It is what it is."

"No miracle?"

"Look," I said, "have you ever watched a ski jumping event during the Winter Olympics? I've seen guys fly 800 feet or more and land so smooth you'd think they'd just stepped off the curb. Same thing with back-country extreme skiing. If the angle is right, a guy can drop almost straight down off a huge mountain cliff, and then he can pop right up from the snow like nothing happened. Bill Jacobs hit the perfect pitch. He landed a perfect ten."

A female reporter I'd never seen managed to push past Jackson.

"Is Reverend Jacobs a prophet?" she demanded. "Should the world listen to what he has to say?"

"That's not my call," I replied. "People can think whatever they want. I came out here only because I wanted to set the record straight on this San Francisco thing. Pastor Gilford was saying some horrible stuff that wasn't true."

Gilford wormed himself back in front of a mic.

"Mark," he said, "you left the prayer meeting at the church to go buy liquor." He swung his arm around to aim his Bible at the big sign behind us.

"Not liquor," I corrected. "Craft beer."

"According to this sign, it appears you have already decided to find your escape in the vices of this wicked world." He raised his Bible towards the clouds. "Ultimate escape, though, is only found in the Lord."

"The Lord didn't paint that sign. You did."

"Nonetheless...."

"I'm not looking for escape." I glanced around. Reporters were holding their questions, waiting to see where this would go. "As far as I'm concerned," I added, "I don't need to escape. The world is just fine."

"Not for much longer," said Gilford. "Not even for you...."

"Pastor Gilford," shouted a new voice from the side. "Do *you* have any predictions that you would like to share?"

"The Bible," he said, shifting into pulpit mode, "is very clear about the End Times. For anyone who cares to read it, the Bible has all of the answers. It also warns us about the false doctrines of demons and the false prophets who will...."

"Hold it," I said, trying to loosen my knuckles. "Be careful before you call Reverend Jacobs a false anything. I find it very ironic that while you're out here talking with television reporters, Freak is inside your church trying to talk with God. If I had to pick who was false... and if I had to guess who was the real deal...."

"You *do* have to pick." Gilford was suddenly in my face. "You *must* decide."

"This isn't about me, pastor."

"It most certainly is. It's about each one of us." He looked at the nearest camera.

"Every person has got to choose."

NIGHTLY NEWS

"Too bad you forgot the beer." Steve zippered his camera bag and pushed it beneath his junk food buffet atop the coffee table.

"Room service can bring us more Killian's from the lounge." I fluffed a couch pillow and swung my feet up next to a bowl of chips.

"Not the same thing," complained Steve. "After all of your talk about those Dillon Beach labels, I really had my heart set on seeing a couple of those."

I found the flat screen remote and boosted the volume.

Saundra had bailed from our convoy to hook up with the Channel 5 mobile unit. They were scrambling, working together up to the very last minute to edit their lead story for their five o'clock broadcast, only a few minutes away. Steve had surrendered all of his footage and returned to the Elkhead Lodge with Freak and me. He needed to be handy on the long shot that anything new might develop on our end.

Now Steve waited with the rest of the world, anxious to see how his Wednesday afternoon efforts would play on the nightly news.

Freak emerged from his upstairs bedroom and leaned down over the lacquered log balcony rail.

"Have you guys ordered yet?" he asked. "I could really use a sandwich or something."

"It's on the way," I called back, popping the cap on another bottle of Irish Red. "Vegetable soup. Beef Stroganoff. Mashed potatoes and garlic toast. Tonight's lodge special. You can chow down with us in front of the five o'clock news."

"Thanks." He disappeared back into his room to make yet another call on the new phone Agent Wilcox had procured for him. Wilcox and Sheriff Andy were presently huddled in the adjacent game room, discussing strategies, spreading stuff out on the pool table, and making numerous phone calls themselves. They seemed to be enjoying their war games, shuttling information and plans up and down their various lines of command.

My own phone was on the nightstand beside my bed, abandoned, still pregnant with dozens of unheard messages nagging for my time. Outdated pleas. It didn't help my motivation any knowing that Wilcox's men had probably already downloaded and screened everything of any possible interest.

Five minutes to five, one of the phones rang in the game room. "Mark," shouted Wilcox. "Dinner's on the way up. Get the door for them, okay? We'll be out in a few minutes."

I flipped the deadbolt and ushered a dark man in a white smock to where we wanted the room service cart—in front of the television, a short stretch between Steve's seat and mine. The man's servant-boy demeanor and his affected English accent were embarrassingly cliché, but his skills with a bottle opener were impressive, and I tipped him first class, signing it onto the room's tab.

On the hour, Freak joined us. Within another minute, Saundra's lovely-but-somber HD visage had also entered our room, warmly but soberly addressing us all from the big screen. Wilcox and Andy pulled stools over from the bar and positioned themselves to take notes from the peanut gallery.

The Summit County disaster epic opened, then progressed in three movements.

Saundra led with a quick recap and update on the global story, followed by the local twist of Freak's survival. The second segment briefly covered the morning's events, including the government's escort of Freak to my cabin, as well as our hike up to the desecrated ponderosa pine.

True to her promise, Saundra limited the footage of Freak to a few quick shots from his good side. She flashed several fleeting frames of the bloody stuff at the tree, then lingered on the pine's skinned bark and scrawled curse only long enough for viewers to catch the message. She discretely mentioned the voodoo doll and horse head, then closed with a brief comment.

No mention was made of the Devil.

"Amazing," sighed Steve. "I guess the producer wants to save the rest of my footage for a weekend in-depth special."

The third segment belonged to Tom Jackson. It was utterly sensational… in the worst sense of the word.

Not bound to Saundra's covenant, Jackson showed little to no restraint in airing shots of Freak's face, nor in spinning events for maximum shock. Footage of Freak in his orange parka—coming and going between the military Humvees and the chapel—was accompanied by a voiceover from Pastor Rodney Gilford, who blatantly insinuated the entire episode may have been intentionally orchestrated by Team Freak as a media event to boost his "Final Hour" television show ratings.

Images of Freak weeping, zoomed tight, scars aglow, were provided courtesy of the True Blue Bible pastor's camera phone. For additional color, Gilford editorialized once again about his colleague's request for oil, as well as the celebrity's bizarre New Age methods of prayer. Jackson ran several bites from the liquor store-church parking lot interview, including a clip of me pitted against the Bible-waving Gilford. It came off as an almost comedic apologetic for the church's "Escape" sign, in front of which we had passionately squared off.

Gilford was shown clutching his black King James, opposite of me, clenching my knuckles white.

They ran my line about Saundra saying Freak had prayed to God, crying for the Lord to show mercy on the people of San Francisco.

Jackson stood alone at the end, mic in hand, pointing at the church's billboard where it leaned against the bus.

Perhaps as payment to Gilford in exchange for the camera phone footage featuring Freak's scars, Jackson ended his segment by paraphrasing the Blue Bible cleric:

"As for the integrity and the motives of Reverend Jacobs—and as for the fate of San Francisco—let the viewer decide. Each of us must choose what we will reject... and what we will choose to believe."

By the time the High-5-at-Five crew cut to their first commercial break, stunned silence had overtaken our room.

I added to the thickness of the moment by hitting the mute.

I glanced around, checking faces. Fussing around with my dinner toast.

"Wow," I finally piped. "This garlic bread has really got some zest."

Freak cleared his throat.

"I'll grant Pastor Gilford this much... he's got courage."

"He's an idiot," I said. "Did you hear what he said about San Francisco... and what he said about you?"

"Well, actually, God is still in control. The Lord used that pastor to set the table. And the Spirit used you, Mark, to elevate the message. Thank you."

"What in the world are you talking about?"

"Pastor Gilford declared emphatically, without soft coating it, that we all have to choose. Tom Jackson repeated the line again in his closing. It will get repeated over and over from now to the end. This is a word from the Lord."

"Good grief."

"Mark, the pastor believes in a living God... but Rodney Gilford is frightened. His ministry and his health have been in decline. He doesn't understand the power of the Lord as anything other than ancient stories from his Bible. Tomorrow, though, he will. The healing power of the Lord will be declared for all who have ears to hear."

Wilcox leaned forward from the stool behind the couch. "Are you saying Gilford's cancer will be healed?"

"Yes," said Freak. "The tumors are dissolving even as we speak. I think Rodney already knows. But it will be confirmed by his oncologist in the morning."

"Baloney," I said. "If that twerp ever had cancer in the first place, you didn't cure it just by starting to say some prayer you never even finished. That's not the way things work...."

"Mark," said Freak. "It is God who heals, not me. I'm only an instrument. Despite your diplomas, it is you who still has a lot to learn about how things work. And what makes you think I didn't finish my prayer for Pastor Gilford?"

"Right. And did you finish praying for San Francisco, too? I suppose that if seven million people wake up without cancer tomorrow morning in the Bay Area, then you'll take credit for the safety and wellbeing of those people as well."

"Stop it, Mark."

"Sure, you've got plenty of patience for Gilford and San Francisco," I observed, "but not so much for me."

Freak placed his plate aside, stood, and addressed us all.

"Okay," he said, ignoring me. "It has begun."

He took a couple steps, then turned back.

"I'm going to my room to collect myself and pray. When I come back, let's channel surf a bit and get a better take on how some of the other stations and networks are handling the story. By comparison, Channel 5 may have let us off fairly easy."

Suddenly, Freak trembled, staggered slightly, then caught his balance on the back of one of the leather chairs. He looked pale.

"Are you okay?" I started to get up, then hesitated as he regained his composure.

"I'm okay," he said.

He closed his eyes for a moment, then opened them at me.

"Actually," he said, "I'm not okay. I'm a mess." He wobbled back to the couch and slumped down. "I'm exhausted. You have no idea what's been going on this week in the spiritual realm. And inside of my head...."

Wilcox cleared his throat. "Bill, maybe we should get you back to the hospital. With the help of an IV or two, or maybe the right combination of medications...."

Freak turned to Wilcox with an odd stare.

He shifted his gaze back to me and Steve.

"Guys," he said. "It's going to get bad. I called my wife an hour ago. I told Ellen to pack up the kids and leave the city yet tonight."

"Are you worried," asked Steve "about the media? Are you afraid after tonight's news, they'll track her down again and harass her with more questions?"

"Not just that. But that, too."

"What's up," I asked.

"Listen, all of you," said Freak. "If you have family or know anybody in San Francisco, call them and tell them to get out. My administrative pastor has put it on our church web site, and it's on the prayer chain. But I don't know who will believe and act if I am not there myself telling them. Most of our television crew says they're staying, because they want to get footage and to help with the communications side of things. But Ellen has agreed to pack right away."

Wilcox cleared his throat a second time. "Are they going to drive... did you tell your wife to come to Denver?"

"Yes. I told Ellen to immediately get the kids as far from San Francisco as possible. To drive at least as far as Reno before she stops for a motel. I'm hoping she can make it to Salt Lake City tomorrow night, and I'm expecting her to be here in Colorado by Friday night."

"I'm sorry," Wilcox apologized. "I don't know if we can cover this for you. I'd have to clear any expenses for gas and motels through my boss...."

Freak looked embarrassed. "Well, I was thinking...."

"Let me cover it," I said.

"What?" asked Freak.

"They're going to need meals, too," I said. "Family road trips can get expensive."

I pulled out my billfold and selected a seldom-used Platinum Visa.

"No," objected Freak. "We can manage this...."

"Remove your wallet," I demanded.

I pointed my Visa at him as if it was a gun.

"I know you're famous, Freak. But I also know you're not rich. One of your critics claims your television show has lost a lot of money. I saw a clip of your family and your old minivan... and your house. I'm guessing your credit cards are pretty much maxed out."

He studied me.

"I insist," I added, pretending to cock the trigger. "Show me the credit card you and your wife both like to use the most."

"What are you thinking?"

"A balance transfer. Call it a loan. Let's make it a thousand bucks."

"Can you do that?"

"Of course. That's how I got through college. My mom did it for me all the time."

Freak slowly withdrew his wallet.

I flipped my card over, grabbed my phone, and started to punch in the numbers.

"Give me your card," I said. "This is easy. Minimum payments are practically nothing. With any luck at all, the world will end long before we have to pay this off."

"What," he asked, "if the world keeps going?"

"Then you can pay me back," I said, "when Disney decides to make the movie."

Freak returned at the bottom of the hour, looking refreshed.

As refreshed as a man could look with half his face still missing.

"Feeling better?" I asked.

"Much." He lifted an Elkhead Lodge pen and a pad of logo stationery from his room. "Let's try some other channels. It's time to get out in front of this disaster. I'm ready to take my notes."

"We're still in it with you," said Wilcox. He showed Freak the first page of the pad that he was holding, which was already half full of black scratches. "My boss says Andy and I have got Freak duty for at least another week."

"Overtime City," sighed Andy.

"Is that really necessary?" asked Freak. "Do you both really need to be with me 24-7 like this?"

"You already know the answer," said Wilcox. "If Uncle Sam calls us off... then the world is going to eat you alive. You remember what happened in the hospital parking lot. After tonight, more than ever, a lot of people are going to want a bite of your hide. And I am not talking just about the journalists. At least a few of your worst enemies are probably somewhere very close, even as we speak."

"The cult?" asked Freak.

"Yes," said Wilcox. "Or whatever they are. Preliminary forensics conjecture suggests a strange mixture of several elements. From the tracks, we're thinking at least five men and one woman. They carried a couple of big coolers to the tree. My guys located the spot where the coolers sat and where the blood jars and sacrifices were pulled out. Every aspect of the ritual was carefully thought through and organized. They did their whole dirty business in less than an hour."

"Was this a Wicca thing," asked Freak, "or something else?"

"Here's where it gets weird," said Wilcox. "The site contained evidence of religious elements not usually found alongside each other. For example, my lead investigator says the voodoo doll suggests one type of witchcraft, but the white horse head suggests something completely different. She has never heard of a ritual where a crucified doll was nailed to an animal skull... that sort of thing is not in the books."

"What about the upside down cross carved on the tree?" I asked. "Is that a common sort of curse, or not?"

"Actually, that wasn't a cross. It was a rune... probably the dangling hammer of Thor." Wilcox looked down at his notes. "In Norse paganism, they use that symbol, along with a white mare's head, when they are really trying hard to make a statement. We're thinking at least one person who has a lot of power in this group is bringing in a great deal of ancient Viking folk barbarism. Or maybe elements of neo-Germanic pagan lore."

"Please," said Freak, "keep me informed as soon as you have anything new to share. It will help me to find focus as I pray. The more I can visualize all of this, the better. I need details to defend myself. And to fight back."

"Besides the cult stuff," said Andy, "we've also got plenty of other problems to worry about."

"Like what?" I asked.

"Like the growing chatter... word on the street right now is not at all encouraging."

"What do you mean?" asked Steve.

"Television," said Andy, "has a huge impact. But TV is not the whole show."

"Social media," completed Wilcox. "Blogs. Tweets. Web pages. YouTube clips. News feeds. Emails."

"You're hacking emails on this?" snorted Steve.

"Of course," said Wilcox. "We're talking national security."

"Private cell phone messages?" I added, tossing Wilcox a grin.

"National security..." said Wilcox.

"Right," said Freak. "But let's start with the nightly news. We've already seen what Channel 5 did with the story. Now let's check out a couple other stations. At the top of the hour, we'll focus on the networks. After that, we'll get the take from FOX and CNN."

The tone and range of coverage on the Freak side of the disasters varied immensely. Stories from all nine crash sites were spliced into a larger narrative, an arc of rapidly escalating international tensions and growing paranoia around nearly every facet of the global economy and local community life.

Utilities, train lines, ferries, bus routes... every system was at reduced capacity or operating on high alert. Airlines were providing extremely limited service, and tens of thousands of travelers were still stranded around the world away from home.

A far-right populist backlash was rapidly picking up steam in both America and abroad. Politicians, international celebrities and diverse religious leaders were suddenly all clamoring for an immediate and "total" military response to the weekend's crimes against humanity.

Mosques were in flames in Europe. Roving lynch mobs were reportedly being ignored by the police in Paris.

Political demonstrations were crippling traffic in London and New York.

The Pope joined other world dignitaries in condemning the "despicable acts" of the terrorists as "inhuman regressions" that should rightly call forth an unprecedented solidarity within the civilized world.

One network anchor declared that while countless maneuverings and isolated attacks had for years been leading up to The Day of the Falling Skies, the world was now "witnessing a hybrid of medieval barbarism and religious fascism without its equal in the history of our planet."

The Freak story was treated merely as a human interest distraction on some broadcasts, while others elevated it to preeminence. Wherever Freak was mentioned, Gilford's footage of Freak leaking tears into his scars made the cut, sometimes in a single quick flash, sometimes protracted during a recap or running commentary.

Those of us with notepads jotted observations off and on throughout the night.

Those without notepads tossed observations in from the side.

"Check it out," I hooted. "A mascara commercial. Right after that close-up of Freak."

We ordered more Killian's.

Steve opened another bag of chips, and Reverend Jacobs finally kicked off his shoes and settled in with a small glass of wine.

26 KRISSY

By mid-evening, coverage drifted beyond the big lead stories and deeper into the territory of sidebars and substantive trivia.

That's when I made my splash.

"Hey," shouted Steve. "Is that *her*?"

I blushed. Off screen, and on.

The gorgeous clerk from the Last Stop Liquor store was sweeping me into her towel and kissing me on the cheek.

The direction from which the footage was shot implicated the sagging-pocket geezer with the iPhone at the other end of the aisle. The news anchor confirmed that the old man's video had been posted into a single social media site, then was copied and reposted repeatedly in less than an hour.

"This one has flamed up into an overnight sensation," observed the reporter behind the desk. He paused as the beach-blanket beauty unfurled from my arms. "This scene of Mark Hanson promoting a local craft beer with his mountain-model friend... has now gone viral."

Hmm.

Freak gave me another of his long odd stares.

"While we were praying?" he asked. "That's what you were doing next door... while we were seeking the Lord in prayer?"

"Well, when you put it that way...."

"That's the same chick," said Steve, "from the Dillon beer, right?"

I nodded.

"Man," he said. "If she looks half as good on a label as she does in those tight denims, I can't wait to get my hands on one of those bottles."

Sheriff Andy popped the cap on a fresh Irish Red. "I know her dad," he sighed, loosening his collar. "A good man."

"A toast," laughed Steve, raising a salute. "To a man who threw some really good genes."

"Her shirt?" asked Freak. "I couldn't tell for sure. Ground Zero?"

"That's what it said."

"Interesting." He took a sip of his wine. "Of course," he added, "they got the angels all wrong. The illustration showed cherubs. Renaissance putti. My two angels were mighty warriors. With swords." He swirled his glass. "Not nearly so cute as those two naked little imps."

254

"Her boyfriend created them," I said. "He's got a studio in Frisco."

"What's her name?" asked Freak. "You acted like you knew her."

"We've flirted around a few times. But I've never asked her name."

Freak put down his wine. As far as I could tell, it was still his first glass.

"You've got a problem, son."

His voice grew serious. "How could you not even know her name?" He shook his head. "I thought I saw it before, and now I know for sure. You've got a Dark Rider. A spirit of lust."

"Guilty as charged," I grinned. "Lots of lust. I love lust."

I took another long hit from my bottle.

"And," I added, "I don't see what the problem is. If I had to remember the name of every beautiful woman I ever met, my head would explode."

Andy stood and took a step towards our circle.

"Her name," said Andy, "is Kristen." He wiped his mustache with the back of his hand. "When she was little, I taught Krissy her Bible lessons in Sunday School."

He looked at me. "She was always a bubbly, affectionate little girl."

Steve pointed a candy bar at the screen. "Apparently, she still is."

"Listen," said Andy. "Like I said, I know her father...."

Wilcox's phone interrupted.

He spoke for a minute, then turned to me.

"Someone is in the lobby," said Wilcox. "My man wants to know if he can send her up. She says she's got something for you."

Two minutes later, I flicked the deadbolt and let her in.

"Kristen," I laughed. "We were just talking about you."

"Git owwwwt!" she squealed, dropping two parcels and throwing herself around my neck.

"Mark," she gushed, bending over to retrieve her bags. "You forgot these."

The first bag was soft and light: a stack of Ground Zero T-shirts and a long poster tube.

The second was the surprise: a six-pack of Dark Mama milk stouts, all wrapped cold and tight in a beach towel. The towel landed on the kitchen counter near the door, the six in my hand.

"How did you....?"

"I found them," she giggled. "They were hidden, out of place in the back cooler. Somehow they had gotten lost there behind a couple of cases of Coors."

"Steve!" I called. "Come check these out." I helped Kristen with her coat.

"The last ones in the world," she smiled.

Passing the pack to Steve, I noticed the top was off on one, and the carton rattled a little light in that corner. I pulled out the empty bottle and gave her a questioning look.

"Sorry," she snickered. "Traffic jam on Main Street. I couldn't resist."

I introduced her around to everyone but Andy, who shook her hand and asked about her father. She studied

Freak carefully, awkwardly, then spun herself around the massive suite.

"This place is incredible," she gasped. "I've never been in a lodge condo this expensive before."

"How'd you find it?" I asked.

"The army tanks," she laughed. "A dead give-away."

"Not tanks," I corrected. "They're really just Humvees."

She helped herself to a few chips.

I noticed she was still wearing her Ground Zero shirt, still tucked into her tight jeans. The other guys seemed to notice as well.

Freak didn't seem to mind the image of the yogi in the orange hoodie, because he kept looking at me instead. Kept shaking his head.

"Here," I said, reaching into the stack and tossing him one of the shirts. "Don't say I never gave you anything."

I rifled the other shirts and located an XXL to fling to Steve.

"Wilcox? Andy?" I shoved my arms through the sleeves of an extra-large and tugged it down a couple times to pull out the creases. "Either of you guys want a shirt?"

"Sure," said Wilcox, sticking out his hand to catch. "Not to wear, but as a souvenir."

"I'll pass," said Andy, stroking his brow line and disappearing into the game room.

"What's this?" asked Steve. He picked up the rolled poster, sniffed it, then raised it to his eye like a telescope.

"You're going to love it," I nodded, clearing everything off the coffee table.

Kristen helped Steve pull off the rubber band and spread it out, while I grabbed four bottles to pin down the corners. We all stepped back together to admire the scene.

Steve grabbed the brewery advertising towel from the bar. "Here," he said, passing it to Kristen. "Why don't you and Mark show us that amazing viral pose."

"Pose?" she asked. "You've already been to my web site?"

"Web site?" asked Steve.

Kristen whipped out her cell phone and quickly tapped the screen several times.

"Is this what you're talking about?" She thrust the phone between us. Steve and I gawked in unison.

It was a great shot, one of her selfies from the liquor store. The angle was looking up at arm's length, with me and her wrapped together in the towel. The advertising poster with her bikini-clad likeness—draped in that same towel—was prominently framed behind her.

"Whew," whistled Steve. "Let me just say something, as one pro to another... that is one *heck* of an effective shot."

He took the phone from her hand and lifted the tiny digital gallery frame almost to his nose. "I especially like the way you worked the composition, placing your big smile in the middle. Nice touch... putting Mark's smirk on one side of your face, balanced with your poster model's wink on the other."

Krissy wiggled, then seductively raised a corner of the towel to her neckline, mimicking the pose from the poster.

"Let's try for another," she joked. "Steve, use my camera. You can take the picture this time." She grabbed my arm and drew me back into her folds.

Steve got into it.

He snapped maybe a dozen quick images, then had us move over by the bar. "Hold this," he said, handing Krissy an empty beer. "Slide the bottle above your head against the corner of the wall, like you did against the mast in the poster shot." He moved my hand around her shoulders and positioned it so I was helping her to hold the towel near her heart.

"I'm liking it," he chuckled, shooting away.

Wilcox refolded his Ground Zero shirt and turned back to the news.

"Mark," said Steve. "You're a little too high. Drop your hand another six inches. Good, right there."

That's when Freak scowled and stomped up the stairs to make another phone call from his bedroom. Or to climb into bed with his Bible. Or some such other Freakish thing.

That was also about the time when Saundra opened the door.

"What the...?"

She stood, frozen. One hand still on the knob.

"Busted," whispered Steve.

He quickly lowered the camera phone, slid it onto the counter, and then slinked back into the most sunken hole on the farthest spot of the couch that he could find.

Saundra glared.

REGROUPING

It wasn't just seeing Steve on one knee in the kitchen, shooting pictures of me and Krissy all tangled up like that.

It was her whole day.

The blood. The Devil. Tom Jackson.

Not to mention her embarrassment from the CNN cable news clip she had been forced to sit through with her boss. The one featuring me outside of the church—the part where I attributed to Channel 5 reporter Saundra Paige the dire prediction of a looming San Francisco unspecified catastrophe.

I learned later that journalists tend to frown upon journalists who contribute participatory additions to the stories they've been assigned to cover. My quote managed to produce yet another layer of grief for Saundra, piled higher and deeper over the way she was perceived to be handling her once-in-a-career assignment.

"Seriously?" Saundra accused, drilling past my fluttering eyelids to someplace deep in my brain, a corner that was primal and deep... and still relatively sober.

She shook her head and moved, somewhat unsteadily, towards the stairs to her second floor suite. She made no attempt to even remove her coat.

"Come on," I said, dropping the beach towel and slipping out from around Krissy. "We're just having some fun. It's been a long day for all of us...."

"Whatever."

"Don't be rude," I called. "This is Krissy. From the liquor store. You met her a couple of days ago when you were trying to run me down."

Saundra turned from the second step, steadying herself on the rail.

"I remember Kristen." She stepped back down from the stairs. "Too bad I didn't."

"Didn't what?"

"Run you down."

I laughed. Too loudly.

"Well," I said, "Krissy wants to go to Denver this weekend. She just came by to collect the $200 reward you owe her for information leading to the accostation and skewering of Mark Hanson."

"In your dreams," snapped Saundra. She let go of the handrail and tilted in my direction. "After everything that happened today, you make me have to come home to this nonsense… in the *kitchen*?" She swung her hand towards the door to my bedroom. "Next time, get a room."

Krissy brushed past me and grabbed Saundra's hand.

"This is soooo cool," said Krissy, finally letting go. "When I told everybody I knew Mark, and that Saundra Paige had come by the store to interview me, they all said, 'no way.' But then, when they all saw me on the *news* tonight…."

Saundra somehow managed a thin smile.

"And now," continued Krissy, "here I am, shaking your hand, right in your own room. And I've met Freak. And Mark has been so nice…."

"See," I said. "No big deal. Saundra, sit down. Let me get you something to drink. Have you eaten?"

Thankfully, Saundra had already eaten, because the service cart was down to crusted plates, and the chip bowl was down to salty crumbs. Based upon the booze on her breath, Saundra had not only already eaten, but had also managed to find time for plenty to drink.

She got as far as the couches, then wavered. There, stretched out on the coffee table, was the bikini poster, still pinned beneath four Krissy labeled Dark Mama beers.

"Okay," she sighed, glancing back and forth between me and Steve. "Maybe we can talk in the morning." She turned from the table and started back towards the stairs.

She stopped when she came to Krissy. She shook Krissy's hand for the second time in two minutes.

"Nice seeing you again, Kristen."

She pointed back at the poster. "And again."

She pointed at a bottle. "And again." She began counting with her fingers. "And again… and again…."

"Rude," I said. "Just because you've had a rough day, don't take it out on Krissy. It's not her fault." I looked around the room, then spotted Agent Wilcox.

"If you've got to blame somebody," I said, "blame him."

"Agent Wilcox?"

"He didn't technically do anything wrong," I said. "But none of us did. But at least he's getting paid five hundred bucks a day to put up with all this drama."

I stroked my chin.

"Hmm," I added. "How much are *you* getting paid, Saundra?" I snickered. "Now that I think about it... Krissy and I might be the only two innocent amateurs in this whole operation."

"Innocent?" challenged Saundra.

Wilcox rose from his chair.

"Okay," he said, crossing the room and putting a hand on my shoulder. "Mark, it's been a long day, and you've had a lot to drink. But that's no excuse. Now you're getting rude, too."

"Too?" said Saundra.

"Rude?" I brushed his hand from my shoulder.

"It's getting late," said Wilcox. "Maybe we should all call it a day and go to bed."

Saundra sniffled. "Fine," she said, turning to me and Krissy. "Everybody go off to bed. But you two need to try to keep it down. I've got to get some sleep."

"Saundra..." I asked, more roughly than I had intended, "How did you end up with the breast bed in Breckenridge? What are you even doing here?"

"Best," she corrected. "The *best* bread in Breckenridge." She caught herself and tried again. "I've got the ... best ... bed ...."

"That's what I'm saying," I interrupted. "How did you get into my digs in the first place?"

"Idiot," she sighed. "You begged me to come."

It took me a few moments, but I finally remembered that she was right.

"Well," I said. "That was before I knew you."

Saundra glared. She crossed and uncrossed her arms, swaying. She seemed to be having a hard time finding a workable way to tuck them together in a way where they'd stay put.

"Too much to drink?" I asked. "Maybe you should have gone home with the rest of your *other* team. You could have all passed out together on somebody else's rug."

"*Yeow*," said Krissy, giving a little shimmy. "Is it my fault that you two are fighting?"

"Of course not," I said. "Saundra is tired and drunk. She's not like this all of the time. Only when the cameras are off."

"For the record," slurred Saundra, "I almost lost this story today. I had to fight like hell to limit the footage on Freak. And then Tom Jackson shoots the whole wad and steals the show. And then you tell the entire planet that I'm the one who fingered San Francisco. My boss is this close to...."

A phone rang in the other room.

Krissy tugged her shirt. "I'm starting to feel kinda awkward. Would it be okay if I just go home now?"

Andy, phone in hand, walked over to Wilcox.

"Someone else is in the lobby," he said, loud enough to quiet the room.

"Who?" asked Wilcox.

"Another friend of Mark's. It's supposedly urgent."

"Drunk... or sober?" Wilcox shot me a glance. "Should we be worried?"

"They checked her out," said Andy. "They said she's good."

I gulped, trying to dislodge from my throat a pretty good guess.

A couple minutes later, I slipped the deadbolt and opened the door.

"Heather," I cried. "What a pleasant surprise!"

I probably should have returned one of Heather's text messages. Or maybe one of the more recent phone calls from my mother.

As it turned out, the two fine ladies had gotten themselves pretty worked up by my many non-responses to their calls. They compared notes and filled in the white spaces with countless frightening possibilities. After several rounds of discussion, it was determined that Heather should call in sick for Thursday and drive up from Denver to personally ascertain the state of my being.

Her instincts as a pre-school teacher had kicked in. She wanted to do an assessment of my health, my mind, and my nap-time sleeping arrangements.

Based upon what I could infer between Heather's nervous laughs, arm slugs and sobs, she had become obsessively concerned about certain Saundra Paige rumors, as well as Krissy towel entanglements she'd glimpsed on television. And, more so, on the Internet. And—during her drive up—certain aspects of my recent adventures that had made it onto talk radio.

In a strange way, this was all good, because it brought to light that Heather had been suppressing irrational fears for several months. For some reason, she suspected I had another girlfriend, or two, perhaps one of whom shared a key to the cabin.

Mom, on the other hand, was less concerned about my naps than she was about what was happening on the playground. She was extremely agitated about how it might look to her friends that I was picking fights on a prime-time news show with a man of the cloth... who was only half my weight.

In front of such a quaint white chapel.

With a steeple.

None of this, of course, was at all clear at the time when Heather stepped in through the door with her favorite yellow daisy daypack slung over her coat.

As I led her towards the others, her gaze flew straight past me to Krissy and Saundra. By the time we started doing introductions around the coffee table, her eyes had fallen to the big beach poster and the four Krissy labels.

What had become a long day, and an even longer night, was suddenly and mercifully cut short.

"Oh..." she said.

Heather reached for one of the bottles. She bumped it instead. It happened to be the only open bottle on the table, and the spill and the ensuing foaming mess across the poster was decisive, if not divisive.

"Oops," she added.

With the help of Agent Wilcox—and the suddenly conspicuous presence of Sheriff Andy's dark uniform—we all quickly came to see the wisdom of completing the remainder of our amazing conversations after a night of rest and detoxification.

Sleeping arrangements became blatantly obvious, with Kristen promptly packing home to her own apartment. Saundra stormed upstairs to her master suite in the loft, door slamming to let us know when she had safely arrived.

And Heather settled, still seething, beneath the enormous comforter on my king-size bed.

With me on the far wing of the living room sectional.

Perpendicular to the snoring Steve.

28

ISSUES OVER
AN OMELET

"Mark... you've got issues."

Freak paused, checking my face for clues, watching to see if I'd take the bait.

"Of course," I said, gulping two more aspirin with the last swallow of my juice. "I confess. I do have issues."

I rolled my head and cracked my neck.

"But I prefer to call them... 'challenges.' And I've got some big ones today. First, this hangover."

I touched my forehead with the empty tumbler in a mock salute.

"And, second, what am I going to do if Saundra and Heather both decide to join me for breakfast... at the very same time."

I lowered the pulp-speckled glass to the table, then reached again for my plate.

Someone, probably Andy, had removed the drenched bikini poster and had wiped the tabletop dry. The empty Krissy bottles had presumably gone the same way as the soggy advertising sign. Hopefully, though, the remaining full bottles had not been tossed out with the empties. In another eight hours, I might be ready to try again.

The thick jade drapes still veiled the entire stretch of main floor windows, but the brilliant morning sun flooded through the huge upper glass panes. Steve managed to pull a cushion over his head and to snore through the sunrise. My night of tossing and my morning's headache were such that only coffee, food and pharmaceuticals could blunt the blades now prodding my skull.

I glanced around the living area, thankful I only had to contend with Freak. To finish my breakfast with him.

As angry as Heather had gotten last night, it was too early to risk carrying my plate through *that* door for my final few bites.

"Challenges," said Freak, "can change from day to day. I'm talking about on-going problems. Things that shadow you 24-7, haunting you wherever you go. In addition to your many daily challenges, you've got much bigger issues."

"So do *you*, Freak." I leaned forward. "If a person is alive, then he's got issues. If he's dead... well, then...."

"We all die," sighed Freak, tapping his spoon against his cup. "And, yes... I confess, I have my issues, too. Right now, though, we're talking about *your* issues."

"Are we?"

I lifted my fork and steered it towards the final vestiges of my omelet. Freak waited, so I continued, assessing my ratio of pepper to cheddar and eggs.

"Maybe," I reflected, "if a person is dead, then the issues are limited to three options. A smile. A scream. Or nothing."

"You," said Freak, "are a trickster... trying to pull me off the real subject." He leaned back. "Mark Hanson loves to play with smoke and mirrors. Misdirection." He glanced around, like I had done, apparently also wanting to confirm bedroom doors were closed.

"Last night," said Freak, "you got ugly."

He cleared his throat.

"You made a drunken fool of yourself. If last night was the first time this week, I'd let it pass. But there's a pattern. And not only your drinking excesses, but there's the flirting as well. You can come off pretty lewd. You treat women too casually, with no thought for how they might resent being jerked around...."

"You're exaggerating..." I pried at a tidbit of bacon, "and you're also underestimating my charms. I've had to clean up much bigger messes than this before. The ladies will be fine. Women enjoy attention. And there's nothing more flattering than a sincere apology the next day."

"Sincere?"

"Of course. I've perfected the art. I can now actually feel the pain of my ways when I grovel." I clanked my fork across the plate a few times, gathering into a small mound the final elusive nibbles. "Come on, Freak, relax. I'm only kidding."

"This is a heck of a thing to kid about. And I'm not sure you *are* kidding."

"Lighten up. It's all fun and games. Nobody gets hurt."

"How would you know, Mark? Are you paying close enough attention to even guess how they feel when you treat them like they're your own little game pieces?"

Hmm.

I thought of the Krissy bottles I'd shuffled around on the deck Saturday moments before Freak's fall.

"So," I said. "I guess you're an expert on women. I take it you and your wife have a perfect marriage?"

Freak shifted, blinking several times.

"My wife and I have our struggles. Ellen is a good woman. I've already admitted that I have issues. But we're talking about you."

"There you go again, Freak. Who says we're talking about me? You're very good at judging me. Judging the world. I sure hope God is easier on sinners than you are, or all of us are toast." I pointed at the platter of sourdough and jam. Then I swung my finger towards his face. "*Toast.* You, too, my friend."

Freak dabbed his mouth with the linen napkin from his tray.

"Fair enough. I've screwed up some stuff with my wife. And my kids. But the Lord has forgiven me. And I'm working on it. Unlike you, I was painfully aware of what I was doing...."

"Ah-ha!" I cracked. "You're a cheating pervert after all, aren't you?"

I thought it would come off as more funny than it did.

Something odd swept over him. The skin-and-flesh side of Freak's face twitched. He turned away. Started to rise. Settled back into the cushion. Took several deep breaths.

"Whatever you may have heard," he said at last, "that is only one side of the story. And, as I've said, God has forgiven me. And I'm working on it. All three of us are... Ellen, me, and God. We're moving on."

"Da-ang.... That was supposed to be a joke. I haven't heard a thing."

Freak met my eyes, briefly.

"Anyway," he said, talking to my empty glass. "I do like you, Mark. And I believe you and I are supposed to work together. God has important work for us to do. So I'm worried about the way you treat women. And, as you can guess, this is something I know a bit about. I know this could blow up on us. On you."

"Hey," I said. "I really am sorry for... whatever. But I'm young. I'm *not* married. And I don't have kids and a religious television show. For me, it's okay to enjoy the good life a little. To enjoy a woman... a lot." I tried to grin.

"Even for you," he said, "it's not as okay as you think. Your patterns—your habits—these things will come back to haunt you. And you will hurt these women more than you think. Trust me, these are not harmless games."

"I'll settle down when the time comes," I said. "And we're talking about grown women. Single women who know what's up. You're a preacher, you know all about free will. They've got free will, too. They get to make the call about what they do or don't do with me."

"You're good at this, Mark. You're a player. I'm guessing at least some of the time, it's more your call than theirs. Some women probably don't have much of a chance when you start putting on your best moves."

"You give me too much credit. I'm doing good if I can bat .500 a season."

"How many women have you slept with, Mark? How many have you dropped? How are you ever going to settle down with only one woman after a decade of the games you've become addicted to playing?"

"I'm not addicted. I'm just making the most of my time. What about you, how many women have you been with?"

He dropped his fierce gaze back to my pulp-stained glass.

"If I didn't believe," he grimaced, "that you and I are supposed to be yoked, then I'd handle this conversation quite differently. As it is, I'm going to say this much."

He met my eyes. "Too many. I've been with too many women. And that's how I know you've given yourself over to something that's going bite you in the shorts. And there will be casualties before it's over, some of the women...."

"How many?" I asked again.

"I'm not sure." He pressed fingers against his temples. "I'm not sure how to even count them. Once we allow Satan to start hanging out in the deep parts of our souls, and once we give him so much working space within our lifestyles, things go from bad to worse in a hurry. The enemy creates strongholds, positions from which he strikes out into other areas of our lives...."

"I'm not into the Devil—I don't believe Satan even exists."

"You should. He's got strongholds on you right now. And it's only going to be getting worse."

"I've got it under control," I snapped. "Listen, Freak, I'm not into perverse stuff. I don't hit on minors. And I don't mess around with married women."

"You know darn well Kristen already has a boyfriend."

For some reason, I pictured Krissy. My heart began to race. Her half-naked beach poster....

"Girls like Krissy," I smirked, "they always have boyfriends. It is only a question of whether you want to wait your turn... or if you're willing to cut in line."

Freak closed his eyes.

"You should hear yourself," he sighed. "There is so much beauty around you... and so much ugly inside."

"No kidding," I said, nodding towards the closed doors. "So much beauty...."

He shook his head. "Ironically, prior to last night, all three of them may have had at least an ounce of respect for you."

"Three?" I twiddled my fork. "The way I remember, you went to bed before Heather...."

"Stop. I know what happened with Heather. You were foolish... but also loud."

"Last night," I conceded, "was not pretty. But like I said, I'm sure we'll smooth it all out. They'll understand. Not that there's anything to understand."

I reached for a piece of toast. "And, by the way, everything was going hunky-dory, and I was in full control of myself last night until you started messing with my head. It was you and *your* issues that derailed the good-times train."

"Oh?"

"You got on my case for not knowing Krissy's name."

"An honest mistake, I'm sure."

"Freak, I let it slide at the time. It might have seemed like I blew it off as no big deal. But you said something... and it really ticked me off."

"What?"

"You said I was demon possessed."

Freak met my eyes.

"You accused me," I said, my voice dropping, "of having a *Dark Rider*. In fact, you said as much in the hospital the first time we ever talked, before you even knew me. I'm not stupid. I know what you meant about a spirit of lust. In fact, I know a heck of a lot more than I sometimes let on."

"Do you know," he asked, "the difference between demonic attachments and demonic possessions?"

I didn't answer.

"I didn't say you are demon possessed. It might seem like it's just language, but language shapes ideas. Vocabulary can shape emotions... even culture."

"Freak, I'm an English teacher. Tell me something I don't know."

"Take the word 'idol,'" he continued. "If the only time we ever use the word is when we're talking about ancient religions, then the meaning seems clear. An idol is something most modern Americans find absurd, like a carved chunk of soapstone nobody in his right mind would ever worship. On the other hand...."

"Yes," I interrupted. "But if you put idolatry on television and give it a patriotic name, then the ratings will go through the roof. Call it *American Idol,* and millions of people will commit to weekly rituals, sacrificing time and money to pay it homage."

I smugly shook my head. "You're forgetting I teach this stuff to freshmen in Mass Media 101."

He took another sip from his coffee.

"For over a decade," he said, "millions of Americans were being conditioned to pick up their phones and to vote for their favorite 'idol.' America's relationship to the *word* idol—and to the concept of idolatry—was subtly shifting. Selecting the idol of one's choice became a celebrated activity. Under the illusion of casting their vote, people were subconsciously acquiescing into a posture of...."

"This," I smirked, "is pretty heady stuff from a TV preacher."

"Perhaps," grinned Freak. "Maybe, like you, I know more than I sometimes let on." He sighed. "Then again, maybe you got me off track again."

"You give television way too much credit," I said. "It was just a show."

"No, Mark. *You* give television too much credit. Television is nothing. I'm talking about the malicious forces behind the curtain. Demons who strategically attach—or even possess—many of those every-day people who...."

"Here we go," I sighed.

"Then you already *do* know the difference?"

"Fine. Tell me. What's the difference between demonic attachments and demonic possessions? You say tomato, I say salsa."

"Mark," sighed Freak, "you are a funny guy."

"Thank you." I licked my fingers from the last of the toast. "That means a lot to me."

"I didn't mean it as a compliment."

"Neither did I."

We studied each other, testing each other's silence and resolve.

"Every once in a while," Freak said at last, "I think I understand why God chose you to be my witness." He shook his head. "And then I don't. Sometimes... you really confuse me."

I added another splash of vanilla cream to my coffee, then stirred.

"On the first day we met," I said, "Sheriff Andy gave me some good advice. Now I pass the wisdom along to you."

"And....?"

I blew a whiff of steam from my cup, then took a sip.

"Freak... get used to it."

He waited until I'd returned my cup to the coaster.

"Listen, Mark. Are you even at all interested in learning about evil spirits, or are we just making small talk here?"

"I suppose I can humor you...."

"Humor me?" He shook his head. "In the Bible, there's this place in 2 Corinthians 2:11, where Paul says demons are always trying to outwit us. But, he says, people who follow Jesus are aware of those schemes."

"People," I said, "who followed Jesus... they should have been less worried about demons and more worried about the Caesars. Roman leaders turned naïve Christians into garden torches. Centurions were the ones who transformed innocent martyrs into catnip in the lion pits. There is no need to blame mythological demons."

"Perhaps," he said. "Then again, maybe the Caesars were unwittingly part of Satan's demonic schemes all along."

"Naturally." I shook my head. "How can a person even argue with logic like that?"

Freak stiffened. "Mark, I don't think your problem is with me. Your problem is with God."

"Wrong. I don't believe in God. *You*, I have seen. My problem is with you."

"Well," sighed Freak. "Then I'm sorry." He hesitated. "You've got a love-hate relationship with me, don't you?"

I gave it some thought. Glanced at the breakfast cart. Searched for the right words."

"Freak," I said at last, "you're a puzzle. You intrigue me. This whole thing intrigues me. But you're right. I'm not sure to what extent I can trust you."

"Trust me? Or trust God?"

"To hear you talk, a guy might think the two are the same thing."

Freak scoffed. "Hardly. I try to listen to God, and to do and to repeat whatever the Lord says. But I'm fumbling. I'm fighting my own demons. Who knows how I might be getting parts of this wrong."

"The fallen angel parts?"

"No, not those. About the demonic stuff... I am sure."

"Freak, now you're scaring me again. Do you honestly believe God saved you from an exploding airplane so you could revive the ancient fear of invisible spirits?"

"No. Not to fear them. But to be aware. One important part of my assignment is to restore a biblical view of reality. To expose the Devil... and all his works."

"First Saundra," I said, "now me. Pretty soon, you will have the whole world seeing demons under every bush. You're going to undo the past thousand years of science to push us back to religious bigotry and superstitions. Is that where we are heading?"

"Of course not. But let me say again, Christians were once aware. They understood the nature of demons. Today, most people are sitting ducks, fumbling along as victims of demonic schemes and spiritual attacks... without a clue."

"Okay, fine. I'm asking. Tell me about those demonic whatevers. Give me a clue. Explain to me about those nasty schemes to steal my soul."

DARK RIDERS

29

"Demons are real," said Freak. "I've had experiences. Not like in Hollywood, but the real thing. Like in the Bible. And like yesterday at the tree."

Hmm. Time for another slug of coffee.

"Before Adam and Eve, and even before he made the Earth, God created the angels. And angels never die. Hundreds of millions of them. Eventually, some of them turned wicked."

He watched my eyes.

"*Paradise Lost*," I sighed. "I've taught Milton for years. It's a hackneyed recycling of ancient pagan myths."

"Read it again," retorted Freak. "Only this time, try to pay better attention to the angel Raphael. Milton put him in there for guys like you."

I shrugged, acting as if I knew Raphael's lines and judged them as inconsequential.

"Of course," said Freak, "Milton had good cause to reference pagan lore. That red dragon and his legions have been everywhere throughout history. Virtually every society has experienced these ungodly powers, and until recently, most of us have taken these dangerous and corrupting spirits quite seriously."

"Too seriously, perhaps?"

Freak glanced again at each of the closed bedroom doors. I glanced at the bathroom door, suddenly aware I'd been drinking a lot of coffee.

"Demons," he said, "are not what people think. They're smart, and they're real. They can influence thoughts and culture far more than most of us dare to admit."

"What's new?" I said. "I learned this much reading comic books as a kid."

"Which ones?"

"You know, the one with the cute pudgy demon in a diaper. *Hot Stuff*, the red devil." I stroked my chin and glanced again at the bathroom door. "Or, maybe I'm confusing Hot Stuff with Casper the Friendly Ghost."

"Exactly! Demons have managed to brainwash us into believing spiritual beings are nothing but a childish joke. A comic from the funny pages."

"So," I said, "you're saying demons hijacked their own identity. Like they did with the word *idol*. And now they have begun rebranding themselves into something silly."

"No. Not begun. Finished. They've completed the job of remaking their image into something absurd to the modern mind."

"Then," I sighed, feigning disappointment, "I guess I should stop looking under every bush for a diapered red cherub with horns."

"Nor should you be looking for a thin man in red tights with a pitchfork and goatee. Those foolish images, and most of the other stereotypes for evil spirits... are worse than useless. They are dangerous. They lull us to sleep. We need to think about demons in a completely fresh way."

"Such as?"

"Think of them as bizarre alien parasites from an episode of Star Trek."

"I think I saw that one," I said, "A classic. Or, instead of calling them alien parasites, we could use Freak's own special name for them. Dark Riders."

"Correct. With the term 'Dark Riders,' perhaps we'll get past the silliness and restore a bit of clarity to a very serious threat."

"I'll bet your preacher pals get nervous when you start changing the language of the Bible."

I reached for my empty glass. It reminded me of a toilet bowl.

"Worse yet," I added, rolling the glass between my hands, "I'll bet you are really ticking off a lot of those naughty little buggers. No... wait. Are they little, or not? How many of them do you suppose can dance on the head of a pin?"

Freak sighed. "It was a legitimate question in the Middle Ages, and it remains so today. It's a question of whether or not spirits occupy space when they cross into our known physical dimensions...."

"Right. They can appear in all sizes. Whatever they want. And if you say they don't wear diapers or red tights, then what *do* they wear when they're out and about?"

I placed the juice tumbler on top of my head. "Do Dark Riders wear fashionable transparent derbies, or do they prefer crystal helmets when they fly off for their dangerous missions?"

Freak reached up and pulled the glass from my hand.

"No hats," he said. "And, yes I've angered more than a few Dark Riders in the past week. One in particular."

"There you go again, pushing my buttons." I snatched back my empty tumbler. "You know how I feel about my germs. These are mine. If you want bacteria, go get another glass. Then pour some juice and grow your own."

I leaned over and returned it to the service cart. The tumbler, along with its semi-transparent orange residue, was now out of the game. So were the teeming hordes of dangerous, invisible microorganisms.

"Listen," he said, his voice flat. "I can understand why you don't want to believe what you can't see. But sometimes... things defy explanation. True things."

"Show me a demon. Show me a Dark Rider. And then I will follow you to ends of the earth. Until then...."

"It's not so easy. They get to decide when they'll be seen... or if they'll be seen at all. Sometimes, they are like shadows. And it's a matter of light."

"Very convenient for them. And for you."

"It is not a matter of convenience," said Freak. "It is a matter of truth."

"Which is it? A matter of light, or a matter of truth?"

"Both. Light and truth are often the same thing."

"Fine. Turn on the lights and tell me the truth. Are there any Dark Riders here right now, or are we alone and safe?"

"Do you really want to know?"

"Of course!"

"Well then... yes."

He nodded. "One that I've ticked off is here right now... a Dark Rider who has known you for a long time. Inside, and out. His name is Lust, and he has been harassing you throughout this entire conversation."

"And here I thought it was the coffee."

"Coffee, yes. Dark Rider... also, *yes.*"

I knew it was a trick, but I found myself squirming anyway.

"How close?" I asked.

"Very close. Within an arm's reach."

"Where?"

"Swirling—orbiting through your head."

"Okay...." I said, drawing back. "Let's forget I ever asked. It's bad enough that you tricked Saundra into seeing angels and spooks. Now you're filling my head...."

"I'm not the one filling your head. This is between you and him. It was you who opened the door."

"I didn't open it to *that.*"

I stared at Freak. Dared him. Begged him. Waited.

"Yes," he said at last. "It was you who opened the door to the Dark Riders. You gave them access. And now you have a chance to undo the damage. To throw them out, and to cut them off."

"Them? Oh, boy. Now you're saying I've got more than one. Multiple demons, *inside...* right now...."

"Not exactly. It's complicated."

"Fine. Keep it simple. Fun and simple. Stick to Lust."

I crossed my legs against the growing burn of coffee and juice.

"You've got a textbook case."

"Sure, it's a textbook case," I said, "because every man faces this same thing. If you want to personify libido and call it a demon, fine. But if it wasn't for lust, the human race would have gone extinct a hundred thousand years ago. Lust is simply another name for love. For life. For putting up with a woman even when half the time you can't stand half of the things she says or does."

I took advantage of the silence to listen. Was rewarded. Another snore from Steve's nest on the couch.

He wasn't eavesdropping.

But then I heard something else. Someone at the door.

"Let me get that," I said, rising to my feet. "With any luck, it's room service with another case of beer. Or maybe the mailman with one of those lust magazines I ordered yesterday while you were hunkered down in your morning prayers."

Freak shook his head as I made my way to the locks.

"Good morning," frowned the stranger.

He stood shifting, gray at the temples, fidgeting in a heavy open jacket with a thick laptop computer tucked beneath one arm. His other hand wobbled up, found itself latched onto a thin dark tie, tugged twice, then dropped back to his side.

"Morning," I said. "Who do you need?"

"Mark Hanson, yes? No? Wilcox sent me. May I sit down?"

I eyed him up and over.

"It depends," I said. "If Wilcox sent you, then what's the password?"

"Password?"

"Just as I thought." I cleared my throat. "You gotta go back and tell Agent Wilcox I don't talk to nobody who doesn't know the password. He should know that by now."

"What in the world are you talking about?"

"Wilcox will know. Now git."

I shut the door and turned the bolt, then headed back to my conversation with Freak.

"Mark, you're clever," said Freak, watching as I returned to my seat. "But you're not very wise. What if Wilcox sent that man up here for something important?"

"What could be more important than this discussion? When it comes to examining my libido, I'm all ears. Well, not all ears, but you know what I mean."

"Do you seriously believe," sighed Freak, "that you can boil all of your lady issues down to something as simple as libido? What about the ways you sometimes feel powerfully driven beyond your own reasonable needs? And the ways you later feel ashamed, conned... even violated by what you supposed were your own actions?"

"There shouldn't be," I said, "any shame in being a robust man. Blame the shame on churches. And meddling mothers. Sure, my attraction to beautiful women and my desire to get them naked drives me to act a bit crazy sometimes. If that makes me a textbook case for lust, then I'm guilty of being a healthy male. A textbook case—with issues—as charged."

"Smoke and mirrors. Mark, what exactly do you want from me? I'm getting some conflicting messages from you."

I drew a long breath, then exhaled slowly. I glanced from door to door, making sure yet again that none of them had opened.

I recrossed my legs.

"Two more minutes," I said. "We'll discuss this for a few more minutes. Then never again."

I let my gaze slide and settle into Freak's scar. As always, the ridges and gouges glowed in an unnerving rainbow of dark reds, purples and pinks. I moved back to his expectant eyes.

"This fallen angel," I asked. "The Dark Rider you say has been screwing me up with women. Is Lust really its name.... is it really here right now? I don't see how one demon can terrorize every man on the planet at the same time."

"Yes, it's here. But, no, its name isn't actually 'Lust.' But if we call it by the name Lust, then the filthy spirit knows he's in the crosshairs. Knows he has been caught in his crimes. Knows he can no longer hide."

"Here?" I asked, waving an open hand around my head. "Or here?" I pointed a finger into my ear. "Where exactly are we talking about?"

"As I said, it's complicated."

"I get it. But now's your chance to fix your broken wingman. To upgrade your witness." I softened my voice. "Tell me what I need to know about this Dark Rider you call Lust."

"Lust is a relatively recent word, so that's not really his name. The particular parasitic organism that has attached itself to you dates to before Adam. And he's only one of a vast horde with the same nasty specialty. But, like every sailor on a ship, every Dark Rider has his own ancient individual name, unique to each creature... going back to the Fall."

"*Right.*"

"Mark, you pretend to be aloof. But deep down, your inner-man senses the frightening truth. Your spirit knows you are not alone."

He leaned close. "I'm here, breathing into your face. But, beyond your immediate senses, you can feel the truth of the presence of two women who are sleeping between their sheets in nearby rooms. The doors are closed. You can't see them. But you sense they are there."

I could.

Freak never should have mentioned the ladies between their sheets. I had to blink a couple times and force myself to stick with our conversation.

"And..." he said, leaning back, "you also know that a Dark Rider is haunting your brain. Right now. If you try, you can sense him as easily as you can sense the women in the other rooms. And you know he's messing with you, because he plays your hypothalamus like an electric fiddle."

"My *hypothalamus?*"

"Yes. It's only about the size of a pea, but it's role in your brain and nervous system can hardly be overstated. The hypothalamus is hot-wired into glands, and it ends up influencing everything from your blood and heart rate to your interest and performance in...." He tossed his head towards Heather's closed door. "Your hypothalamus directly effects what happens between the sheets."

"So maybe some of us are pea-brained after all?"

"In your case," Freak grinned, "without a doubt."

"So where do Dark Riders fit into all of this?"

"You let your Lust Rider hang out with you. Most of the time, you appreciate his little surprises... you enjoy what he does for you and your body. At strategic moments, your Lust Rider sends very tiny pulses of energy into a critical spot on your hypothalamus. A few pin-prick surges can be enough to siderail anyone who is unaware... or anyone who is uninterested in fighting back."

"Spiritual warfare?"

"Yes, in one of its many forms. Think of how a single well-placed spark can quickly flare into a raging forest fire. From glands to hormones... and then to your nervous and circulatory systems. Shooting like flames through your body in a matter of moments. It's frightening what an itty-bitty well-placed surge can do to a man's entire system."

"Sure," I snorted, "I've felt the flames. But I'm not blaming demons...."

"Of course not. And he'd like to keep it that way."

"I heard a preacher say God created sex to be mind-blowing. We're supposed to be able to enjoy a partner."

"Absolutely. Don't hear me wrong. There is something spectacular and worth singing about in the way God made our minds and bodies to work. But who is in charge? You? Or...."

"And you think you can see this Dark Rider, right?"

"Picture this, Mark. You awaken in your tent. It's in the black of night. Gnats are buzzing around your ears, brushing against your nose and lips. You swipe your hand right through the swarm, but they're still there. You're afraid you might breathe some into your mouth. Gnats...."

"Time for the bug spray."

"But *Mark*... how would you know where to point the can?" Humans put way too much stock in our eyes."

"But you keep acting like you can see them."

"Sometimes everything is a blur. Sometimes, not as much."

"Well, you said I've got one right now. My gnatty little Mr. Lust must be growing nervous. Angry. He hears you trash talking him, so he is probably turning red... huh?"

Freak straightened. Closed his eyes. Opened them slowly, focusing above my brow.

"Yes," said Freak. "Your Rider is agitated. Angry at me. At this very moment, I sense an energy that you might call red, although it is a stretch to assign it a color."

Freak closed his eyelids. Then he lifted one hand as if he was suddenly seeing more clearly.

"Right now, your Rider is slipping in and out, spinning around your head like an electric vapor...."

I coughed. "An electric vapor?"

"Yes, a pulsing, red vaporous energy...."

"Or," I cracked, "perhaps I should be looking for a swarm of fire ants with tiny beating gnat wings?"

I abruptly stood.

"This is crazy," I said. "I feel like I'm sitting with a gypsy in a carnival side show."

I stepped around the coffee table and headed towards the common bathroom on the main floor.

"Thanks for the mixed metaphors," I called over my shoulder. "But my gland-of-the-hour needs attending, and that comes first."

30
STEAMED

I could hear the hissing water jets of the steam shower deep within.

Freak had returned to his room. Over my shoulder, Steve snored on.

Otherwise, I was alone.

"Heather," I softly called again. "All of my clean clothes are on your side of the door."

I didn't need to be tricked by some Dark Rider.

It had been almost two weeks since I'd been with a woman, and my own natural unashamed hormones provided plenty sufficient drive to energize my circulatory system and to keep me moving in Heather's direction. And I didn't need to apologize for anything.

I quietly opened the unlocked outer door and slipped into the small living area of the main floor master suite.

Her yellow floral daypack was on my bed, along with a pair of her slacks and my favorite flannel shirt. The clothes she'd worn last night while driving up from Denver were strewn across the floor. Her coat was draped from the back of the swivel chair at the desk.

I crossed the living space and entered the sleeping area, then approached the closed bathroom door.

"Heather," I called again, more softly than before. I began unbuttoning my shirt.

Whatever her flaws, and she had several, I kept picturing how she'd look when I joined her in the shower.

The images had filled my head and quickened my pulse ever since I'd heard her enter the shower several minutes before.

"Honey," I said, testing the knob. It turned easily. Was also unlocked.

Inviting.

I gently pushed open the frosted glass door and stepped into the steam-filled granite tiled room.

"Heather...."

She screamed.

Loudly.

"It's me," I shouted back, making sure she could hear me over the spraying water. "It's just Mark."

"Get out!" she screamed again.

"But...."

"Out!"

Five minutes later, she finally turned off the jets.

Meanwhile, I abandoned my shower fantasies and simply swapped the clothes I'd slept in for a clean set from the dresser... after four quick sprays of cologne. Then I sat on the bed and waited. Watching the door. Trying to remember if I'd left the short white lodge terrycloth robe still on the hook inside her door.

Hoping I hadn't.

It took her another five minutes to finally emerge. Fully robed, almost down to her knees.

"What the hell," she said. She seemed surprised to see me. She cinched the robe even tighter.

"Heather," I said. "The door was unlocked. I took that as an invitation. Back home, whenever...."

"This is not back home." She flicked her hand at me, motioning for me to shoo from the bed and go sit at the desk.

"But this is my room," I complained, slowly rising from the bed. "Dang, Heather, you look good when you're mad. With wet hair."

Her legs were perfectly tanned, no small feat given that flip-flop season was still several months away.

She yanked yet again on the white terry belt.

"You've got a lot of nerve," she said. She moved neither towards her clothes on the bed, nor towards me. "What's been going on up here? I drove all the way over the Divide last night, worried half to death. And then I find you in this plush palace, with those other two women...."

"Nothing happened," I said.

I removed her jacket from the chair and piled it onto to the desktop, then sat.

"Look," I apologized. "I'm really sorry about how it might have looked to you last night when you arrived."

"It didn't look good."

"But think about it, Heather. If I was sleeping with either of those other two women, do you think I would be so eager to slip into the shower with you this morning...."

That didn't come out right. I caught it.

Thankfully, Heather did not.

"Mark," she sighed, finally stepping in my direction. "I haven't known what to think. First you blast out of town without me. And then, all of a sudden, you're on the news...."

"Yes," I said, reaching for her hand. "It's been crazy. You have no idea."

"No, I do have an idea." She halted, one stride short of my grasp. "Everybody knows something is going on. This stuff about you and that disfigured man is everywhere on TV. Every day. Practically every hour."

"You can't believe everything you see on television."

"Did that *man*..." she asked, "did the preacher really fall at your cabin? Did you actually see him land in that horrid tree?"

"Believe it or not, I did."

"It must have been awful. Digging him out from the deep snow and everything."

"Yes," I sighed. "It was a real nightmare. I think I'm still in a bit of shock."

"Well," she said. "I would imagine."

"Thank God," I said, "that you're here now to help me pull myself together. But how did you find me?"

"Those two big army tanks. I was driving around, and I spotted them right away. Even in the dark."

"Not army tanks," I corrected. "Military tactical vehicles. They're basically just overweight Hummers. Lots of people seem to make that mistake."

"Oh...."

"By the way, how was your drive up?"

"Okay. I suppose. The Denver radio shows would not stop talking about *him*." She stepped away and lowered herself onto the nearest edge of the bed.

"Is it true," she asked, "that the preacher wants everyone to call him Freak? Is that what you call him?"

"I guess. I know it sounds strange at first, but after a while, it becomes like a regular name. In fact, most of the time, it's gotten so that I hardly even notice his scars."

"His scars...." Heather shuddered. "Where is he staying? I suppose he's staying somewhere here at this same lodge?"

"Actually," I said, "I'll introduce you later this morning. His bedroom is at the top of the stairs...."

"What!" She jumped to her feet.

"It's really not a big deal," I hastened. "He's not that bad of a guy...."

"Was he here... last night? While I was sleeping? Why didn't you tell me he was staying here with us in this same room?"

She shivered, then sat again on the bed.

"Hey," I said, standing, stepping towards her, spreading out my hands. "This place is huge. It's like a hotel within a hotel. He's not sleeping anywhere near our room. We've got our own suite, and he has a place of his own. He is not even sleeping on the same floor as us."

"Us?"

"Look," I said, placing my hand on her shoulder. "If you don't want to meet him, you don't have to. Like I said, this place is huge."

Heather shrugged off my hand.

"I need to get dressed," she said, standing. "And you need to leave. We can talk after breakfast."

"I've already eaten. But let me order you a big fancy tray from room service... whatever you want. After you've eaten, you and I can take a walk. Then we can get caught up and talk this all out."

"Well... okay. But it sure would have been nice if you had found a few minutes to call me this week. I started to believe you weren't even thinking about me."

"I was thinking about you, Heather." I met her eyes. "Honestly."

The rest of the honest truth was that I had also been thinking about Saundra. And Krissy. Wondering what might have happened if Heather hadn't driven up... or if Krissy might have stayed until she was too drunk to drive home. Wondering what might have happened if—instead of Heather—I had walked in on Krissy in the shower.

I became aware of a bizarre sensation, as if electric gnats were buzzing—ever so quietly—within my ears.

"Okay," said Heather. "Order something healthy for me. No meat. And then we can take a walk and try to figure this all out."

I tentatively stretched my hand down to hers.

She took it, then gave it a soft squeeze. I leaned and planted a quick peck on her cheek.

She pulled back slightly, then dropped my hand.

"I need to get ready," she said. "Now get out."

31
VILLAGE WALK

While waiting for Heather, I flipped through the newspaper tabloid that appeared each day from under our door.

Still more questions than answers about the airplane disasters.

Another less-than-convincing promise of resolution from the President.

Increasing speculation on the potentially catastrophic repercussions looming over the months ahead.

More sweeps and arrests. Isolated outbreaks of chaos in the Middle East.

A headline story from a group in Iran complaining about the cowardly use of drones against innocent children and sheep.

On page eight, a full-length feature on Freak.

According to the story, a fan base of sorts was developing on the Internet.

Blogs were lighting up.

Meanwhile, strong opposition to Freak's message and character was calcifying among coalitions of influential church dignitaries and political celebrities.

Fringe groups were floating absurd statements into the mix, presumably just eager to see their names and ideologies in print.

By scanning for direct quotes, I got the sense fans and foes alike were more excited about what Freak had said in years past—and what they expected him to say in the near future—than anything he had actually said during the time I had known him.

Heather pushed her empty plate across the counter.

"Let's get out of here, Mark. That man," she nodded towards the top of the stairs, "knowing he's up there makes me really uncomfortable."

"Sure," I said, putting the paper down. "Let's go. Let's take our walk and get some fresh air."

"You're not listening," she said. "What I meant was... let's go *home*. Back to Denver. If you're still worried about being chased by all of the reporters, then you can spend the rest of the weekend over at my apartment with me. The reporters won't even know where you are."

I stood from my stool.

"It'll be okay," I said. "Things will work out. They always do. Let's get outside first. Then we can decide what to do once we clear our heads with some fresh air."

"But," she protested, "you need to be back at work on Monday. I don't understand why you decided to stay here with him in the first place. And why are you letting that television lady sleep here, and all of those other guys who are always around...."

Steve lifted himself from the couch to his feet and shook his leg.

"Okaaaay," he said. "I can see it's time for me to check in with my boss upstairs. Some of us guys and gals are on the clock. Some of us have to work for a living. Despite appearances, we're just doing our jobs."

"I'm sorry, Steve," said Heather, slipping from her stool. "I didn't mean it the way it sounded. But while I was alone in my apartment back in Denver, I was worried sick. I didn't know what was going on up here, and I was trying day and night to get Mark to answer his phone. And come to find out, he was here eating and drinking the whole time. Sitting in this fancy lodge with a bunch of big-shot strangers, and...."

"Heather," I said. "I've already explained this. My phone was at the cabin."

"Why couldn't you borrow a cell phone from Wilchuck? Or from the policeman?"

"*Wilcox*," I said. "And the other man's name is Deputy Sheriff Andy Dekkers. Technically, there is a lot of difference between a police officer and a county sheriff deputy...."

"There you go again," she said, pulling away. "Why is it that you always have to correct me about every teeny-weeny thing I ever say wrong?"

"Steve," I said. "You don't need to leave. Heather and I will go. We'll continue this conversation outside. We'll both cool down, and everything will be fine."

I turned back to Heather.

"I'm sorry," I said. "You're absolutely right. These past few days have been very confusing. I've been a jerk. Let's take our walk. And if we both agree it's time to leave, then we'll pack up and go."

"Really?"

We entered the lobby and knew immediately something was wrong.

One of the many new security men from the Wilcox team stepped from the conference room doorway and moved toward our elevator door as soon as it opened.

Looking past the plainclothes agent, I could see through the lobby windows and glass doors where a mixed mob was milling about. They were arguing with the hapless lodge staff and with security.

And apparently with each other.

Only half of the crowd carried cameras or notepads, the others preferring torches and pitchforks. Several brandished primitive signs on sticks with misspelled placards expressing various three-to-five word opinions, mostly stated as demands.

In classic form, one of the signs read: "REPENT! The End is Near."

I stopped to study the scene while the suited Wilcox man gathered speed in my direction.

"Sorry Mark," he said, lifting a hand several steps away. He leveled his arm towards my chest, as if preparing for a joust. "Are you trying to leave the premises?"

"Yes," I snapped, more agitated by the man's thrusting cuff-linked limb than by the barbarians at the gate. "What's going on?"

"As you know," he replied, "we have strict orders. Nobody has cleared you for leaving this morning. I'll have to call...."

"No problem," I said. "I'll clear myself. Thanks for your concern."

I took another step, but his arm grew stiffer.

"You can't just leave," he said.

"Whatever," I said, brushing past his arm. Heather followed in reluctant tow.

He grabbed my arm from behind, and a second stranger, this one in uniform, quickly blocked our path in more definitive terms.

I shook the first man's grip from my arm.

"What the heck," I complained. "What's going on?"

"Trouble," said the uniform. "And the protocols for dealing with troubles."

The stranger turned to Heather. "I'm sorry, Miss Nickleson, but we're going to have to get this cleared before we can let you go any further." He reached for the small black two-way com device clipped to his collar."

"How," I demanded, "do you know our names?"

"You're Mark Hanson," said the agent, exaggerating his impatience. "You're the Denver high school teacher who pulled *him* from the snow. You're staying with *him*, along with Agent Wilcox and Deputy Dekker. Plus you've got a cameraman and Miss Heather." He nodded politely in my damsel's direction. "Additionally... there are two other women who have been cleared to stay with you as well."

"Right," I demanded again. "I don't have Alzheimer's."

I glanced at Heather. She was knotting an eyebrow, perhaps visualizing big x's through the two unnamed women from the agent's list.

"My question," I said, more annoyed than ever, "was, how do you know me? And who gave you orders to stop us?"

He shrugged, as if speaking to a child.

"Mark, if anyone on our team didn't already know your face from the daily briefings, they would at least know who you are from the television news." He lifted his chin. "It was Wilcox—and his boss—who told us that nobody comes or goes without a prearranged clearance."

He nodded towards a desk ten steps to the right.

A dark agent leaned our way from a high stool perch. He sat eyeing us like a vulture, with tiny fidgeting concierge shuddering below, nearly swallowed within the dark bird's shadow.

"That is Agent Wright. He's in charge here on the ground floor. Our orders are for every person who comes or goes to be checked through him."

"Fine," I swore. "Let's go meet Mr. Wright."

Before we reached the station, I had already begun my irate and indignant fuss about being restricted—detained unconstitutionally, and now humiliated....

Only to be rudely interrupted by a loud thump.

I glanced over to the glass entrance. Several bodies jerked and thrashed in a brief scuffle.

The establishment made short work of the insurrection. A densely-bearded mahogany man in a green jacket was whisked away, feet dragging, yelling something

I could not understand. He quickly disappeared in the direction opposite of the lodge's effectively secured front entrance.

Facing inwards from where he'd dropped it against the thick glass door was a bright poster-board sign.

"SMILE..." read the top line of the hand-scrawled quip. "GOD LOVES YOU."

Dominating from the bull's-eye center of the message was a huge, universally familiar yellow icon, but with a rather unhappy face. The poor fellow's smile was upside down, and crocodile tears flew in all directions from plunging eyebrows and squinting eyes.

The sign's creative surprise was plastered on the left side of the yellow face.

A florescent pink patch covered the cheek, presumably placed there to represent bad acne... or perhaps a fallen prophet's supernaturally acquired scar.

I had no idea whether the message bearer was a clever friend, a crazy fiend, or a sane foe. And I didn't have a clue as to the meaning of his enigmatic little missive.

Within moments, the sign was snatched up in a blur, perhaps to be re-borne by a cohort, or maybe to be delivered into the incendiary fires of the Summit County landfill.

"As I was saying," I continued, turning back to Agent Wright, "would you like us to fill out some paperwork? Thank God for protocols...."

Agent Wright momentarily conferred remotely with Agent Wilcox. Together, they quickly developed an appropriate written plan. In triplicate. Reasonable for the most part, signatures not-withstanding.

They clipped onto each of our collars a small high-tech two way radio device. We were instructed how to activate communications if we encountered any more God-Loves-You rowdies.

Busloads of unregistered knuckle-dragging activists had begun arriving from around the compass, apparently loosely organized by disparate apocalyptic blogs and zombie flash mob visionaries.

I requested a self-defense taser, but was denied.

"Let's get you out through a back door," said Agent Wright. "There's no sense running the pretty lady through the front door gauntlet if we don't have to. Without a gun, I'm not sure even I could make it out alive."

Heather and I were turned over to another two agents. We were eventually led down a gloomy service hallway to an inconspicuous sunken loading dock in a dingy back nook of the lodge complex. We managed to avoid knocking our ankles and shins against vegetable crates and stained milk pallets, and then were given directions for weaving through four green dumpsters in order to merge with a wooded bicycle trail on the west side of the lodge. From there, we could follow the path all the way into town.

The tallest uniform made a final security offer to accompany us for our entire walk.

No thanks. Have a nice day.

Smiley face.

Free at last.

The air was crisp. Warm in the high-altitude sunshine, cool and brisk when sauntering in the shade of the pine and ski village shadows.

Groundskeepers had long since cleared the winding streets and meandering bikeways, including our trail that linked the Elkhead Lodge to the rest of the town.

We strolled past restaurants, through shops and in the lee of tall condos and hotels. Only occasionally did we have to catch ourselves in small patches of black ice.

I slid my hand into Heather's as we crossed the slick spots, then slipped it out easily when our walk again turned bright and dry on the far side of a shadowed crossings. Together, we ignored events of the past few days, recalling instead our last mountain getaway. Our last romantic meal. Our last weekend at her apartment.

I reached deep, drawing from my well of significantly convincing enthusiasms to add to our remembrances; Heather's cheeks bloomed pink in the cold, her bare hands remaining warm between her pocket thrusts and our random boutique dalliances.

"I'm sorry," she said, "about the way I yelled at you in the shower this morning."

"No, that's, okay. I was out of line."

"Were you?"

I had to think about it. Was I, or wasn't I?

"Is something wrong?" I asked.

"Let's go home," she finally sighed, her voice dropping in revived despair. "You're friends up here are all very intimidating."

"I'm sorry," I said, "Wilcox is a total jerk. If it helps, I promise... he's not my friend. In fact, if I get a chance, I'll be sure to punch his nose."

I pointed at the gondola loading station where our path opened wide at the base of the vast white Breckenridge basin.

"Here's an idea," I said, feeling naughty and looking for a way to deviate from our signed Homeland Security recreational itinerary. "What if instead of going home, we rented some skis and caught a few quick runs while the slopes are still sunny and warm?"

The ski lift lines were shorter than I could ever remember for such a perfect spring break day.

Heather considered.

The rental shops, and even the coffee bars, were also more sparsely peopled than I would have expected.

Far up the mountain, above the tree line, only a handful of dark boarders and skiers etched the stark white pitch. The sky, which had begun so hauntingly clear, was beginning to cloud gray.

"No," she said. "The sun is going fast. It's starting to get chilly. I didn't dress for cold. Especially for higher up there, where the skiing is best."

"Listen..." I said, submitting to the powers that be. I began steering us back towards the most direct return route to the lodge. "I've been thinking about some things Freak has been saying. Not just his predictions about more disasters in the world, but some other stuff, too."

"Like what?"

Part of me wanted to tell her about the Dark Riders. But another part of me didn't. Wouldn't. Knew I never would.

"Well," I said, "Freak keeps telling me God saved him by using me. That it is my destiny to work with him... in some crazy way."

I stopped. I faced Heather and took her hands.

"Freak has made a big deal out of the fact I was the world's only witness to his survival—to the miracle of him hitting the tree from an exploding jet. And that I saw with my own eyes the way his shredded face was healed practically overnight."

"Lucky you." She scrunched up her nose. Her little wrinkles weren't as cute as I remembered from when we'd first begun dating several months before. "Did he predict," she continued, "when the rest of his face would be healed? It's pretty disgusting, you know."

I released her hands and resumed our walk.

"Freak asked me," I said, turning a corner and heading up a slight grade. "He begged me to give him a little more time...."

"Then what?"

She grabbed my sleeve and made me again address her eyes. "So what if he's right about the disasters and everything. You saw all of those angry people trying to get into the lodge. What does any of this really have to do with you? I don't think it's even safe to be around him."

Several teenagers were approaching, giggling, bumping into each other's hips.

"The thing is," I said, quietly as I could, "if he is right, then maybe some sort of apocalypse is really coming. Then maybe God is real. Maybe Freak actually has been chosen to share a message for the end times."

I let the young people pass.

"And," I said, knowing how strange it would sound, "maybe God chose me out of all of the people on the planet to be the one who would help Freak to convince the world that...."

"Oh boy."

She shook her head. "I never thought I'd see the day when Mark Hanson took a job in religion. Is that television preacher going to give you your own program, or are you going to be working on his show... aiming a spotlight on him from the balcony or something?"

Hmm.

We walked a block or two in silence. Eventually, we stepped off the sidewalk and back onto the plowed trail to the backside of our lodge.

"Freak wants my help," I said. "I'm going to kick myself the rest of my life if I don't stick it out long enough to know for sure."

"What" she asked, "if I'm scared? What if I don't want to sit around here waiting with you?"

"You're a big girl," I said, kindly. "You have to do what's right for you. I hope you stay, though. This is pretty important stuff."

She took a deep breath. "How long?"

"Through the weekend. And you saw how good the security is. You're probably safer sitting here than you'd be in a Denver jewelry store."

"Sunday?"

"Yes. Maybe we'll know more by Sunday night."

32
BREAKING NEWS

By the time we returned to the lodge and passed through security, the temperature had dropped considerably.

I pushed open the door into our suite, weary, hungry, and cold.

Steve was walking from the kitchen toward the sprawling leather sectional, oblivious to all but the blaring television news feed.

"Yo, Steve," I called, kicking off my boots. "Heather says we should order up some soup...."

"Mark! Where have you been?"

I stepped onto the carpet in my sweat-clinging socks.

"I told you we were...."

"There's been an earthquake. A big one!"

"Where?"

"San Francisco. It's on every station."

He turned back toward the television, moved three steps, then spun around.

"Hi, Heather," he said, tumbling his words. "Sorry to be so abrupt. I hope you had a good walk?"

"I did, I guess." She tried to smile.

"Mark tells me good stuff about you all the time," he lied. "We'll have to talk... later today."

She looked at me, then again at Steve.

"Go ahead," she urged. "Get back to your news. This sounds like quite a big deal."

"It is," he said. "Let's get to know each other this afternoon. And then I want you to give me all the dirt on Mark."

Steve rushed back to his seat. He threw himself into the cushions, then called over his shoulder, changing his voice, addressing me.

"We got the word from Wilcox a few minutes ago. He called up from the lobby and told us to turn on the news. Wilcox will be joining us again here as soon as he finishes with his meetings downstairs."

I moved into the great room and stopped at the outer edge of the couch corral.

Freak leaned toward the enormous television flat screen from the closest spot on the sectional. Sheriff Andy kept shaking his head from several cushions away.

Both were frantically taking notes as new information was added to the loops. Saundra was alone around the corner of the couch at the other end, her stylus flying.

"Mark," said Freak, glancing up briefly as I found a place to stand behind him. "It's hard to believe that while we were talking this morning... it had already begun."

I nodded.

After several moments of news, I stepped away to drag two stools from the bar. I gestured for Heather to join me there in the back row.

Freak was already glued again to the screen. My Ground Zero shirt was under his elbow, wadded where I'd thrown it during my restless night of banishment from my own bed.

"Freak," I said, "there's somebody I want you to meet."

He looked over in time to catch Heather frantically signaling no.

He started to get up, assessed Heather's body language, then sat back down.

"Nice to meet you, Heather," he smiled, turning back to the news.

"You too," said Heather, her face ashen.

News from the Bay Area was bad.

Not utterly catastrophic.

But not at all good.

Several dozen deaths had been immediately confirmed, along with hundreds of injuries. The death toll was expected to rise dramatically throughout the day.

The epicenter had been a few miles southeast of the historic town of Petaluma, almost 40 miles north of San Francisco, on the Rodgers Creek Fault.

The worst of the local devastation was sustained by crumbling historic Victorian structures, many of which had survived the great San Francisco Earthquake of 1906.

Headlines quickly moved from the immediate death toll and the extent of localized damage to broader concerns, including the lack of any hint of forewarning... and the severity of the earthquake, which was felt as far away as Seattle. The event registered a magnitude of 6.8.

Nobody was sure what the morning's disaster might mean for the rest of the Bay Area. Initial comparisons to California's 1989 Loma Prieta "World Series" earthquake were easily made. The biggest difference was that the Petaluma quake was a product of the inland, highly complex Hayward Fault system, rather than the relatively straight-forward and well studied strike-slip coastline movements of the San Andreas.

Scientists could only speculate as to what to expect from aftershocks. They were uncertain whether this quake might trigger subsequent events within the Hayward Fault Zone... or beyond.

The most immediate concern focused on several hazardous Union Pacific and BNSF train derailments, along with two roadway failures in the North Bay industrial district near the East Shore Freeway.

One of the derailments involved several bulk railcars carrying pressurized liquid gas. Their proximity to parked tankers filled with toxic and flammable chemicals created the potential for explosions.

Fears over possible ruptures and major spills were spreading, with rumors of evacuations circulating on the streets. Emergency risk management experts were discussing several frightening scenarios involving the nearby Chevron Richmond Refinery, whose record of chemical leaks and industrial accidents compounded everyone's concern.

BART and other transit services were suspended, pending repairs and inspections throughout the region. The extent of breaks and ruptures among the region's buried water and gas pipelines was still being assessed, and over a million people were without power.

Wilcox soon returned.

He glaringly avoided me.

He strode through the room, then lifted from the floor the empty end of Saundra's sectional unit. He swung it around to face the TV more directly, then took a seat beside her.

The two of them promptly began whispering and comparing notes.

Like the rest of us, Wilcox was apparently trying to get as much information as quickly as possible. He was also paying close attention to how the media handled the tone of each story.

After a while, I noticed Heather ignoring Saundra and everybody else. She sat silent, turning back and forth only between Freak's scar and the glowing screen. She appeared ready to be sick.

Experts disagreed about what might happen next around the Bay Area. Few expected any significant related activity from the San Andreas Fault, but the potential for adjacent multi-fault ruptures, especially within one of the densely-populated cities between Berkeley and San Jose, was apparently on everyone's mind.

"The Northern Calaveras Fault," observed one bespectacled, bald, bearded scientist from the United States Geological Survey, "that is the wild card grabbing my attention at the moment."

"What of the Hayward Fault?" asked the reporter.

"Well, of course, the danger with the Hayward goes without saying. We've known for a long time the North Hayward Fault is fully reloaded. After this morning's event, the clock is now ticking—it is only a matter of time before we see a significant release."

"Reloaded?"

"Strain has been building since the last major Hayward Zone rupture, which was in 1868. The Hayward Fault has a cycle averaging approximately 140 years between major failures. The likelihood of a massive adjustment has increased significantly with a Rodgers event of this magnitude. Some of the best models suggest sequential segments will likely fail in pairs."

"How soon?"

"Days... months. A few years. We have decent models, but we don't have enough specific data yet today to provide any reliable predictions."

"But, as I said, it is the Calaveras Fault we know the least about, and perhaps those are the lines we should be watching...."

Freak lifted the remote and clicked through to another station's coverage.

A public official, hair mussed, jacket open, swayed in a slight breeze before a black bloom of microphones.

"... and because so many of the Bay Area highways run directly atop or alongside fault lines, as with the Warren Freeway in the rift valley at Highway 24, our freeway system is extremely vulnerable. Not just major bridges, like the Oakland Bay Bridge, but numerous other interchanges, viaducts and overpasses. Any of these could fail during a succession of quakes, especially where a compromised structure surviving one event is suddenly pushed beyond its reduced integrity by an immediate second or third event...."

Collapsed warehouses and partially destroyed churches and schools, along with localized urban fires, were providing compelling backdrops for live reports.

Mobile news teams confirmed that several retrofitted transportation and public structures on the east side of San Pablo Bay had suffered disappointing failure, but San Francisco and Oakland had weathered the quake surprisingly well.

Preliminary guesstimates placed total structural losses at 2-4 billion dollars.

"It's not over," sighed Freak, sliding deep into the couch. "Not even close."

Saundra broke her heavy silence.

"Freak," she said, pulling his eyes from the television. "Is this what you saw when you prayed?"

"Yes. And no. We are witnessing only the first pangs."

"First pangs?" asked Steve.

"This is the beginning... of the beginning... of the end."

"Are you saying," asked Saundra, "that you think San Francisco is going to see more damage? I hope you don't honestly believe the rest of the city..."

"Eventually, yes. We are all moving towards closure. Towards the big finish. For California... the end...."

He turned from Saundra to me.

"For America... the end." He dropped his voice.

"And for the world... the end."

Saundra lowered her nose back toward her phone pad. She tapped her stylus once to her upper lip, flipped through a few screens, then feverishly began to write.

"What's next?" she asked.

"Dominoes," said Freak. "North Hayward... South Hayward. Then a catastrophic event from the Calaveras, which will trigger a response from the San Andreas. A response that will exceed the San Francisco earthquake of 1906."

"And...?"

"San Andreas will move later this weekend... major adjustments throughout the entire system, grinding and snapping all the way down to Los Angeles."

Freak watched her frantically scribble.

"Yes," he said. "L.A. will follow the way of San Francisco. And then Seattle and the Pacific Northwest."

When she looked up again, he addressed her, softly, deliberately.

"Of course, Saundra, you may quote me...."

We all waited.

"But," he continued, glancing back at the TV, "I believe it is time to put our favorite Channel 5 News reporter back on the global stage. And back in favor with her boss."

She responded with a questioning look.

"Saundra," he asked, "are you willing to do another interview?"

"How soon?"

"Could you and Steve be ready in an hour?"

"Yes. That could work." She slipped her stylus back into her phone.

"Again," she added, "I am not going to be able to promise you anything live. My producer will be all over this. He will insist upon unconditional freedom again to exercise complete editorial discretion."

Freak nodded consent.

She glanced at Steve, then back at Freak.

"Would you rather," she asked, "that we do the interview here, or...."

"Whatever you think. I trust you."

Wilcox abruptly stood.

"Leaving the lodge right now" he said, "is out of the question. We can control things best from right here. But are you two sure about this? I'm really concerned that as the California death toll keeps rising, the rawness of this disaster on top of those shocking terrorist attacks will make people...."

"I'm sure about this," said Freak. "People need the truth."

"Uh... Freak," said Saundra, looking tentative. "Would you like me to help you with some makeup? It would be very easy for me to tone down the reds...."

"No." He touched two fingers to the flaming gouges of his left cheek. "This interview needs to be me... as is. Real, and raw."

"Why now, Freak?"

"Because... the Lord has cried out through both the rocks and the skies. It is time."

Freak excused himself with his notes to go pray in his room.

Saundra made two quick calls, wished Heather a weak good morning, then dashed upstairs to finish her hair and makeup. And to rethink her wardrobe.

Steve engaged Andy's help in rearranging the room.

He adjusted the lighting and prepared his equipment to shoot Freak and Saundra with the enormous central stone fireplace as a backdrop. Another cameraman from Channel 5 showed up at the door with a tripod and his own pack of equipment, then quickly began coordinating with Steve for another angle while resolving a potential sound issue.

I moved Heather onto the empty couch beside me. I swapped a few observations with Wilcox and Andy, always keeping one fascinated eye upon the news.

"The slip-fault movement," said a consultant from the California Geological Survey, "between the North American Plate and the Pacific Plate is well understood. As a tectonic meta-narrative, we see where our state has been, and where the West Coast is most certainly destined to go. But the variables for locally destructive earthquakes—once a renewal of accelerated shifting begins during a succession of related strain and breaking events—is beyond calculation...."

I bumped up the ladder to the next saved channel option.

Heather excused herself to use the bathroom.

"If," said a well-groomed young man, "we had another major earthquake like the one of 1868, and if it were to occur here, along this fault line," he drew a line with his finger down the length of his map, "then the damage would be nothing less than catastrophic. Over $ 1.5 trillion worth of property exists along this corridor."

He tapped his knuckles to the map.

"This entire corridor would be decimated. An estimated 5 million people would be significantly impacted. An estimated 2.4 million people would be cut off from sewer service and flowing water. Fire fighters and law enforcement, and especially medical personnel... they would all be totally overwhelmed...."

Heather leaned into me from behind the couch, wrapping her arms tightly around my shoulders.

"Do you understand this?" she whispered. "California has had earthquakes before. Why does everybody seem so much more panicked this time?"

"Acting hysterical drives their business," I said. "That's how they keep viewers from switching to a different channel. That's their job... to make it seem like every little thing that happens is the end of the world."

Andy swore.

"*Little* thing?" He waved his hand at the flat screen. "Mark, this is serious stuff. There will be some innocent First Responders who will die before this is over. There will be some chaos tonight... and looting. And if the Bay gets a few bad aftershocks, it will quickly get worse."

"Yes," protested Heather. "But the California reporters on television seem even *more* frightened than they usually act. They keep talking about all of the worst things that could ever possibly happen."

"They are scared," said Wilcox. "And the media is still totally juiced from the Falling Skies Massacre last weekend. For America to experience two unrelated disastrous events like this in less than a week...."

"Shhh...." I interrupted, cranking up the volume.

The footage on the screen featured a fast-flowing montage of numerous Freak clips from the past few days. It opened with his hospital interview and his quote about the impending "death of millions." The voiceover recapped critical backstory on Pastor Bill Jacobs, about his television show called The Final Hour, and his miraculous fall and survival from the terrorist attack.

Then they rolled a few seconds of tape from Freak's unmasking at the hospital, followed by two different exterior orange parka shots. The montage ended with an interior chapel tight zoom, courtesy of Pastor Rodney Gilford. Freak was shown weeping into his scars.

"Reverend Bill Jacobs," said the reporter, "has captured the world's ear. But what is he saying? Is it true that he accurately foresaw this morning's earthquake in California?"

The feed switched to a rerun of me... arguing with Pastor Gilford in the True Blue Bible parking lot.

"I was there," I shouted in the clip. "Saundra said she heard Freak praying *for* the city. Not against it.... Freak wasn't cursing the people of San Francisco, he was crying out for God to show them mercy."

"The question," said the reporter, again filling the screen, "may never be answered. Reverend Jacobs has neither confirmed nor denied his alleged prediction of a San Francisco earthquake. Nor is there any indication he ever suggested a specific date or magnitude of the disaster. At this point—one man, Mark Hanson—claims someone told him Bill Jacobs mentioned San Francisco in a prayer this week."

"That's all we've got, folks. And, of course," concluded the reporter, "vague earthquake predictions for California are a dime a dozen. A person may as well predict that next winter it will snow... in Nome, Alaska."

The reporter rotated toward a different camera.

"In a bit of mixed news, we're getting new information on that rapidly developing weather system currently bulking up over the Pacific. Northern California has been unusually dry for this time of year. In combination with low humidity, this has contributed to the challenge of urban fire containment this morning in the Bay Area. Two inches of rain are expected from this system, which should help with fire mitigation. But with rain will also come an increased risk of landslides, especially in the event of localized heavy downpours or aftershocks."

He turned to back to center.

"More on the weather in three minutes. But first, here to update us on the increasingly fierce battle to contain the derailed tanker fire in Richmond, we have live reporter...."

I hit the mute.

Hmm.

Heather again squeezed my shoulders from behind. She slid her arms back off from her embrace until she was down to just a pair of hands clenching my neck.

"You looked pretty mad on television," she said. "I hope you never yell at me the way you were shouting at that little preacher."

"Of course not," I said.

She let go of my neck. "Mark, let's go home."

"Soon," I replied. "Soon enough."

33
ON THE
RECORD

"Yes," said Freak.

He glanced beyond the improvised fireplace studio set. His eyes rose past Saundra in her chair all the way over to me by the kitchen.

"I know how this may sound," he continued, "but it is the truth. San Francisco is about to be completely destroyed. And the city—San Francisco as everyone in the world knew it up until last week—will never be seen again."

Steve pulled his brow away from the camera viewfinder.

Shook his head.

"Okay," sighed Saundra. "We'll try that question again."

She looked in Steve's direction to confirm he was still filming, even though his head was far from the tiny digital window.

"Freak, as you know," she said, "this is all going to be edited. Go ahead and say whatever you want. Keep in mind, though, that whenever your comments get too far out there like that... I can guarantee you my producer will chop and drop those lines as fast as you can say them. Comments like the one you just made will never make it to the air."

"I know," said Freak. "And all I ask is for *you* to keep in mind that I am not generating this out of my private imagination. Nor am I speaking on behalf of my own agenda. When you and your producer are done cutting this interview, please clean up the floor and file all of the outtakes. Some of what you reject for tonight's broadcast may be of use tomorrow." He winked. "You never can tell."

His arrogance was unnerving.

For a man with only half a face, he had returned from his room after an hour of prayer with a whole lot of nerve.

Freak requested for me to remain at hand throughout the interview. More than a little curious—but a little put out because he'd framed it as a command—I complied.

Heather, Wilcox and Andy were also invited to remain. The four of us non-participants sat together on the stools behind the bar, me with my left hand off and on Heather's right knee, depending upon how agitated she became.

She had not yet adjusted to the disfigurement of Freak's face.

Nor to the horrors she witnessed on the morning's news. Thankfully, Heather had apparently acquired a new phone, and during much of the interview, she seemed content to distract herself trying to figure out her contact list and some of the new apps. I didn't think much of it, knowing her number would still be the same whenever I needed to call.

Freak largely ignored the three beside me; it was only to me his comments occasionally turned. Knowing he was an experienced television professional, and realizing therefore that the attention that he gave to me was intentional, I was all the more annoyed.

"Freak," I called. "At this rate, we'll be here all afternoon. Please focus. I was hoping to use the gondola to get in some skiing before the next earthquake takes out the entire Western Grid."

He smiled. "Thanks for your sense of humor, Mark. We're going to need your quick wit from time to time over the next few months. Otherwise, we might as well slit our wrists right now." He took a sip of water. "Yes, I'm afraid it really is going to get that bad. For me... and for you. And for the entire world in the coming days."

"Reverend Jacobs," said Saundra, recrossing her legs and shifting in her chair. "You've predicted a scenario of widespread destruction along the California coast. What is your projected timeline for these events?"

He hesitated.

"It has begun... and it will continue until the end."

"Do you have any advice for our viewers?"

"Ms. Paige, you've been fishing for something specific. A date. A prophecy to discredit or to validate my position...

a test that the nation and the world can use to determine my reliability to speak on these matters."

"And...?"

"Good Friday."

"Tomorrow?"

"Yes. Until now, the most powerful recorded megathrust earthquake in American history also happened on a Good Friday. God has a thing about earthquakes on Good Friday."

He did not smile.

"The last major Good Friday earthquake was in Alaska, barely over 50 years ago. Tomorrow, California will experience a series of earthquakes that will together make the force and the destruction of the Great Alaskan earthquake pale in comparison. In terms of suffering, tomorrow will be far worse in almost every way imaginable."

Saundra decided to keep the interview moving, to collect on film whatever usable bites she could, and to leave any further censoring and editing in the hands of her producer and the Channel 5 team in the truck.

"My understanding," she said, was that the 1964 Good Friday earthquake occurred in a subduction zone, and it had a magnitude in excess of 9.0."

"Best estimates," said Freak, "place it at around 9.2."

"Surely," she said, "you do not expect anything of that magnitude in California? Given California's tectonic and geological conditions, scientists have speculated that 8.2 is the maximum magnitude possible...."

"Correct. No single event tomorrow will surpass 8.2. But the issue is not merely how hard buildings and systems will shake, but how many times they will be shaken. And for how long. Imagine a car hitting a single big bump. In most cases, the car will be able to limp home for repairs. Now picture the same car hitting a washboard of big bumps in a series of hard jolts. One after another, over and over, until hose clamps finally work loose, delicate electronic systems rattle into dysfunction... and a bumper finally falls from the frame."

"Aftershocks?"

"More than mere aftershocks. We can expect a series of powerful shakings lasting 15 to 60 seconds each. Tomorrow, we can expect a rapid succession of significant quake events, mostly in the 7 range. Man-made structures and landslide-prone embankments that were weakened today will be further traumatized tomorrow by a North Hayward rupture, followed by a powerful South Hayward release. Then everything will be capped tomorrow night by a Great Calaveras earthquake surpassing 8.0, lasting upwards to two minutes without a pause."

"Reverend Jacobs... suddenly you are being *very* specific."

"Please, Ms. Paige. I appreciate your attempt to show me respect on the air. But I must insist yet again for you to address me by the new name the Lord has assigned. Please, call me... Freak."

"Okay... Freak. You are being very specific."

He turned his left cheek more directly towards Steve's camera.

"The Lord has chosen me... and the Lord has marked me as an embodiment of a prophetic message. In this final hour of human history as we've known it, God has called me to speak truth and warnings to America, and to the world."

He slowly turned to the other camera, addressing the stranger behind the tripod personally, yet as a representative of our species.

"We have entered into an hour of mercy. God loves us all, sinner and saint. And the Lord has appointed this hour as a time of invitation. This is our last hour for salvation, and God's final invitation to life."

He turned back to Steve.

"But, also, this is an hour of judgment... and of death. It is time for the world to believe. To repent, and to obey."

Saundra again recrossed her legs.

"Freak," she began, "you mentioned God has marked you...."

"Yes... my scars."

"Why would a loving God leave you with such a disfigurement? Doctors agree that your overnight recovery was a miracle of sorts. If God granted you this miracle, then why did he not finish the healing work? Before your fall, you were a handsome man..."

"Thank you, Ms. Paige..."

"... but now... many people find your appearance unnerving. It is probably not politically correct of me to say so, but your present appearance is certainly not...."

"God makes no mistakes."

He smiled, boldly, deepening the shadows in the troughs of his scars.

"The Lord has saved me. He has appointed for me to carry this face. It is a gift to the world. It is a powerful, embodiment. A visual proclamation of His Word."

"What word is that?" asked Saundra.

"Grace," said Freak. He lightly brushed his right knuckles up and down along the smooth, healthy right side of his face.

"God has called me to share a message of grace...."

She nodded.

"And..." he added, moving his hand to the other side, "I also bring a companion word." He slowly drew two fingers down the glowing ridges of his hardened wounds, down from his temple to his chin. "I bring another word as important as the word of grace."

He tapped his scars.

"I bring the word... of truth."

"Tell us," said Saundra, "what do you mean by the word 'truth.' Please say a bit more about your understanding of God's truth for us today."

"God's truth can be like this scar on my face. It is not always pretty. It can involve pain and suffering. It is a natural consequence of sins and mistakes. Evil men blew up my plane. I fell. My face was disfigured. This is truth."

Once again, he raised two fingers to stroke his shredded and plasticized left cheek.

"The world," he continued, "is broken. It groans beneath the weight of humanity's mistakes... and it shudders in the shadows of the looming, ugly, painful consequences of our sins."

"Freak," said Saundra, "these are harsh, confusing words. Frightening words."

"Ms. Paige, you asked me a while ago what advice I have for those who watch this interview. Let me offer several items."

"First, if you live in the San Francisco Bay area, then you should pray."

He leaned towards the nearest camera.

"Pray... *right now*. And listen to what the Lord has to say. If He tells you to leave, do so immediately, before the bridges and the roads fill with the panicked masses... and before the infrastructures collapse. But if God tells you to stay, then you should prepare immediately."

Freak reached to beside his water glass and gingerly lifted my mother's Bible from the table.

"For those of you who decide to stay in San Francisco, but who are not in a good relationship with the Lord, I urge you to beg the Lord for His forgiveness." He opened the Bible near the middle, then gently caressed the written pages with his free hand. "I encourage you to receive His pardon through Jesus Christ."

"And," he said, removing his hand and closing the book, "I invite you to make the most of this one final opportunity to faithfully obey your Heavenly Father. You must now do that which is valued highly in the Lord's sight."

He opened his empty hand.

"Tomorrow, when that escalating series of ruptures, shakings, and judgments begins... help others."

He gently drew the Bible to his chest.

"Pull them from the rubble. Calm their heart-rending sobs the best you are able. Offer mercy to them... bathe them in loving songs and tender prayers. Bring them water... even as they die."

He returned the Bible to the table and exchanged it for his half-filled glass.

"Life-giving waters," he said, lifting the clear tumbler towards Steve's camera. "Share the waters of love and life... even as they die. Even as *you* die...."

Saundra cleared her throat.

"The Lord," said Freak, looking directly into the camera, "God will give you one last chance to do what is right. To love your neighbors as you love yourselves...."

"Well," said Saundra, straightening in her chair, "I can neither challenge nor vouch for anything you've just shared. What I would like to emphasize, though, is that an overnight mass-exodus of San Francisco is neither possible nor advisable. A complete evacuation...."

Heather nudged me. "Look, she whispered," holding out the phone. "When I zoom in, it's just like we're watching the news. Except the news hasn't even been made yet."

I briefly glanced down at the phone in Heather's hand. I nodded, hoping she would be satisfied and stop talking.

"I agree," said Freak. "Most people should stay in San Francisco... in their own homes, and in their own neighborhoods."

"But," said Saundra, "in your opinion, many of these people will die if they don't evacuate tonight."

"We all must die."

Freak opened his hands. "The entire world will soon face judgments on the order of San Francisco. Southern California is next, and then the Pacific Northwest will follow with a Cascadia subduction event followed by a devastating tsunami. After that, we can expect a wide range of catastrophic events spreading across America and the rest of the world. Some of these disasters will be driven by the sinful nature of man. Others will be so-called natural disasters. But all of them will have supernatural forces behind them. Trying to run away may buy an individual a little time, but it will not reverse the direction history is heading."

He turned again to the other camera.

"For many thousands of Bay Area residents, tomorrow is the appointed day of their death. For the rest, their day of passing from this life will arrive soon enough. Unless the nations repent, the end is at hand, and a world-wide collapse of everything...."

Saundra sighed.

"Look, Freak, you know I won't be able to use what you just said...."

"Keep it," he said. "Maybe later."

"Off the record," she said, glancing at Steve, confirming he was still in a recording mode. "How bad is it going to get tomorrow?"

"On the record," he smiled, nodding at Steve. "Very bad. Everything I said about the earthquakes is true. Systems will fail, and bumpers will rattle loose. But that's not all."

"What else?" she asked.

"Unnecessary horrors."

"What do you mean?"

"Evil... broken, lawless and demon-nudged people..." he answered. "Wickedness will rise tomorrow in an unmistakable riot of hell in the midst of a city's horrible fall. What happens tomorrow will be shown on live television around the world. It will play on screens everywhere as a sign to all of the depravity of humankind.

Of our own natural descent towards anarchy, judgment and death... unless we turn to the Lord."

"During major disasters," objected Saundra, "people in the past have often pulled together. Sometimes human beings are at their best when...."

"Not tomorrow," he said. "A minute ago, I described how a washboard of jolts can rattle apart a car. The same thing can be true of our minds... and of our humanity. Tomorrow, thousands of people who are spiritually fragile and emotionally ungrounded will be rattled and shaken until they snap."

Freak's voice was sad and soft, but firm.

"This weekend... San Francisco will shake until it becomes a madhouse... and the Devil will dance among the ruins."

34
OFF THE RECORD

"If the world is going to end," I joked, addressing Steve, "then I say we should all pile into the Humvees and head for the nearest mini-mart."

Freak stood with a fresh glass of water beside Andy, who quietly stared at me, starched in his dark uniform at the far end of the kitchen bar. Saundra was outside in the parking lot, busily negotiating with her producer in the Channel 5 truck. Sifting for usable clips from the morning's controversial gloom-and-doom recordings.

"Let's empty the junk food aisle," I continued. "Let's clear the shelves of the potato chips and every bag of candy we can find. And then, after the power grid goes down, we can torch the place to keep warm."

"Don't forget to grab some comic books and glossy magazines." Steve smirked. He clinked my bottle from the facing stool. "Why not? We can toss them onto the fire as we go."

"In your opinion," I asked, "do you think Saundra will want to join us in our binge?"

"Maybe," laughed Steve. "It all depends upon how today's work plays on tonight's news."

"Hmm," I hummed, taking another drink. "I forgot about the liquor store. We're going to want to load up right away, before the looting and shooting starts. After lunch, let's go find a case of 20-year-old Scotch... and a couple of cases of champagne for the ladies...."

Heather rolled her eyes.

"Right," she said, putting her sandwich down beside her soup bowl and taking another sip directly from her third bottle. "What makes you think you're the only ones who like Scotch? If Freak is right about the future, then I think it is time to hit the hard stuff... for all of us."

Freak shook his head.

"Or...." said Freak, turning towards the stairs to go up to make more calls from his room, "perhaps instead of getting drunk... we all could fall down on our knees and pray."

"Naw," I said. "It's probably too late for a prayer meeting. I say... let's party."

He spun, facing me, more angry than I'd yet seen.

"Brace yourself, Mark. We're talking about God's eternal judgment and wrath. He is fed up with that sort of attitude and behavior. God is starting to call in America's

IOU's for holiness. By this time tomorrow, you'll know what I mean. The whole world will."

"Turn or burn, right?" I snapped.

"Yes. Repent or perish. You're no dummy. You've read Luke 13:5. You know what's at stake here."

"Whatever happened," I said, "to 'God is love'? I thought God loves us just the way we are."

"It is Satan who loves you just the way you are," retorted Freak. "Yes, God loves you, but he also wants to change you. To make you more like Jesus."

"Whatever."

Freak shook his head. "It's time to get with the program, Mark."

"This is your deal," I said. "I say you're just mad because room service brought you ham and cheese instead of...."

"Knock it off, Mark. This is *not* a joke. God has put things in motion...."

"You and God can do whatever you want. I didn't sign up for any of this."

Steve and Heather slipped from their stools and headed with their bottles back to the couch.

"Wrong," said Freak, pointing at my face. "When you were born, you decided to cry and to start breathing. You signed the line. Thirty-some years later, every time you breathe, you sign that line again. You say to God... I'm still in this."

"Fine," I said, "then I guess it's time I opted out." I made a clown show of plugging my nose and puffing out my cheeks.

"Right," said Freak. He folded his arms and waited.

After a few moments, I spurted a laugh and grabbed a few quick gulps of air to get caught up.

"So," said Freak, "I guess you decided to opt back in?"

"Instinct," I said. "My involuntary reflex is not the same thing as willfully agreeing with God about anything...."

"You are not a tree stump or a rock, son. You have consciousness. You have a free will, and you are making life-and-death choices. This is between you and God, whether you openly embrace the truth or not. It is a moral choice—with consequences—when a man chooses to live a self-centered life of willful denial."

"So you say." I finished my bottle and slapped it down on the kitchen bar with a clank, not sure what else to do.

Thankfully, someone began pounding at the door. I figured it had to be another agent from the Wilcox team, maybe even the guy with the laptop that I'd brushed off the other day with the password ploy. But I needed an excuse to catch some air, so I headed back to the locks.

It was Tom Jackson. With his own cameraman.

Rolling.

"Mr. Hanson," rushed Tom, swishing a mic in my direction, "has the prophet Freak made any new predictions?"

Tom was fast and slicker than the laptop man. He was in the room and in my grill before I could either brush him off or bolt the latch.

"Has Freak said anything," he pressed, sliding half way around my side to get himself into the frame, "has he gotten any word from God about the future of California? Or about the timing for the next round of terrorist attacks? About global wars... or the end of the world?"

Tom's feisty cameraman stood much lower than Steve, but his leg was plenty long and quick enough to boot the door shut as he filmed his way into our suite. Sheriff Andy stood firm, apparently recognizing Tom Jackson and willing to see how the scene might play.

"Hey," said Tom, pointing his mic past me toward Freak.

"Hey," called Tom again, his eyes sparkling up another notch as he changed directions mid course. "Reverend Jacobs, we've never been formally introduced."

Tom slithered behind his black microphone like a snake chasing down a dark rodent. "I'm Tom Jackson from Channel Five, and I'd like to ask you a few questions...."

It could have been interesting, but Steve was up and blocking the trail with a raised arm and a "Whoa there big fella!" before Tom ever reached his prey.

And then Saundra was suddenly flinging wide the reckless front door. She pounced on her rogue colleague like a mongoose hunting for a litter of five.

"T.J.!" shouted Saundra. "Who let you in here?"

Tom shrugged my way, then addressed her fury.

"Listen, Sandi, I know this is your story, but...."

"How did you get past security? Does Agent Wilcox know you came waltzing in here without an invitation?"

Tom feigned confusion. "Security?"

"Out! You've got ten seconds, or I'll call Wilcox myself and have him personally escort you all the way back to Denver."

Tom hesitated to the count of six, then briskly made for the exit. Saundra followed him out into the hallway, then slammed the door behind the three of them. Her voice grew distant as she scolded and threatened them both all the way into the elevator, then presumably back downstairs to the lobby and out of the lodge and across the parking lot to their boss in the big truck.

"Now that," I said, grinning at Steve, "was a real disaster."

Steve smiled, looked at Freak, then quickly retreated back into the other room.

"Come on, Freak," I cajoled, slipping back onto my stool. "Where's your sense of humor?"

"Humor?" Freak closed his eyes. "They call what happen last weekend a massacre for a reason. And the tragedy that is about to hit California is beyond anything you can conceive...."

"Oh, don't be so sure. You wouldn't believe some of the movies I've seen. Everything from Planet of the Apes to Zombie Apocalypse. When it comes to epic annihilations, I've got quite the imagination."

"Wise up," threatened Freak. "God intends to use these disasters to open our eyes, to destroy wicked strongholds...."

"Preach it, Rev."

I scowled and dropped from my stool. Andy shifted uncomfortably, looking away. He found a few items on the counter to gather and bring to the sink.

"Mark," said Freak, "God saved me last weekend. And he's working on you today. And next week... God wants to start shaking and saving the world on a scale beyond your wildest imagination."

"Maybe some of us don't *need* to be saved. Or maybe some of us are just willing to save ourselves."

"You can't save yourself any more than I could when I fell from the plane."

It was early, but I stepped over to the refrigerator and pulled out my fourth bottle.

Out of the corner of my eye, I caught a little rustling over on the couch in the other room. An automobile commercial was playing between the Petaluma earthquake updates, and Heather was swinging a pillow at Steve.

"Oops," she giggled. "Sorry 'bout that."

Steve laughed, then grabbed a small couch cushion and swatted his reply.

An empty bottle tipped on the glass tabletop, clanked, rolled, then dropped to the soft carpet at their feet.

"Freak," I said, "thanks for the allegory of the grave. Have a good life." I again started to leave.

"Hold on," he said, almost asking.

"Seriously," I said, stopping. "This has all been way too much fun."

He stepped towards me. Took a deep breath.

Dropped his hand.

"Okay," he sighed. "Let's cool down. You're right...."

"Right about what?"

He found his way to one of the empty stools. Andy started running water in the sink.

"You're right to be frustrated. I've not been very diplomatic." He grinned. "Keep in mind, I did do a face plant from an exploding plane..."

"Don't forget the angels," I said. "Unlike you, I don't have angels singing over me."

He tapped two fingers against his drinking glass.

"You're right. You don't have the advantage of seeing angels...."

"Or demons," I interrupted.

Freak took a deep breath.

"To be completely honest," he said, "I'm not sure if seeing Dark Riders really provides all that much of an advantage."

"*Now* you tell me."

"I'm sorry," he said. "I apologize for being so pushy." He took another huge breath. "Seriously. Just give this one more night."

"Why?"

"Because you're already in it this far. You're standing in the middle of it all—at a critical moment in time—with a prophet who was given a message from God. You've got a front row seat for some of the biggest miracles in history."

"Wow, Freak. You really are a piece of work."

The volume was back up on the television. The commercial was over, and a new live report was coming in from the scene of the tanker fire. Heather and Steve had put down their pillows.

"Miracles?" I asked, picking up my bottle.

"My safe landing was the first one. You saw it yourself. Then the miraculous healing of my face. Pastor Gilford's cancer. And now... my predictions for tomorrow."

I took a few steps towards the couch.

"Another minute," he begged, suddenly soft. "Look, I keep forgetting that if we're going to be friends, I've got to trust you. To trust God."

He stood, glancing toward the TV area, then back at me. "And you need to do some trusting, too. If not God, then at least trust your own eyes."

"You're not making it any easier," I said, "when you keep calling everything some kind of miracle."

He studied my face.

"Mark, the stakes are doubling down even as we speak. I need to be able to count on you. Next to me, you're the most critical person in this mission. God has convicted me that you're a key person in helping to get this faithless dying world to start listening...."

"But," I protested, "you know I don't believe...."

"So you keep saying." He looked pained. "I feel sad—honestly—for guys like you. Guys who think they're too smart for faith."

"Faith is a *private* choice, Freak." My gaze slid from his eyes to the hideous scar. "Dude, it's a free country. We get to believe whatever we want."

"Even if it's not true?"

"Sure. What is truth, anyway? It's all a matter of perspective."

"Tell that to gravity," grinned Freak.

"I think," I said, "Sheriff Andy over there would agree with me." I pointed my bottle at him. "No miracles, right? Am I right, Andy?"

Andy hesitated, glancing between the world's foremost prophet of the sky, and the prophet's faithless wingman, who seemed ready to bail.

"It's all a mystery to me," said Andy. "If you're asking for my opinion, then I'd have to say maybe there are no miracles. Then again, maybe it's all miracles."

I popped the cap from the cold bottle in my hand.

"No miracles," I said, taking a swig and turning back to Freak. "But a world full of opinions."

"Not opinions," said Freak. "Facts. Reality is comprised of truths, each of which is either embraced, ignored, or denied."

"In your opinion."

"Like I said, tell it to gravity." He smiled. "Can't you at least trust me on *that* one?"

I didn't laugh.

"You're wasting your time, Freak. I'm not convinced everything you preachers teach is true."

"No, Mark. What you're saying is that you *are* convinced I'm teaching stuff that is *false*. There is a difference."

He leaned a weary elbow onto the kitchen bar, then ran his fingers through his hair.

"Mark, apparently, you think I'm a fraud... or a fool."

"Hey, I know you're not a fool."

He studied me. "Fraud, then?"

"I didn't mean it that way."

He stiffened. "Okay, I'm hearing you...."

I didn't attempt to reassure him.

"Mark, thanks for putting it on the table. Now I need to hear from the Lord."

"Let me know what you two come up with," I said. "But don't take it personally. You're not the only friend I've got who still believes the Bible. We're adults. You and me can still be friends, even if I don't...."

"Friends?" He threw up his hands.

"Mark, we're talking about the end of the world. Millions of lives are at stake. I need a partner. I need a man who will humbly and passionately serve this cause and go down with me if it comes to that." He turned and walked away.

He didn't even face me when he said it.

"I guess, " he said, "I'm finally realizing I need a dedicated follower... not just another friend."

35 HIGH SCHOOL TRAINING

When I was young, my parents settled me and my two sisters into a Denver suburban church known for its massive indoor gardens and its Disney-class children's ministries.

I grew up among lollipop shepherd dioramas and plastic action figure rewards for quaint little Bible verse regurgitations.

The land of Oz.

Willy Wonka's Chocolate Factory for almost seven years.

And then came high school. The big move from fluff to meaty stuff. From Nestlé's Milk to pepperoni. That's when Pastor Ted took me under his wing, and that's when my religious training took a turn towards the sometimes harder, sadder truths of life... in the real world.

Pastor Ted was by far the most articulate staff member of the youth team. He sported an edgy patch of facial hair. He had a degree in philosophy, and he proudly carried a fresh set of credentials from one of the top seminaries in the country. We all loved him, and it was he who— between ping pong serves and slices of pizza—bumped the arc of my faith development from wobbly sentimentality into a rationally calculated trajectory.

"Keep in mind," he said, eyeing me through his tiny wire-rimmed spectacles, "that every so-called miracle must be properly understood. Past, present, and future.... Palestine, Africa, America, it's all the same. Wherever, and whenever. Physics will always be physics."

He touched the side of his nose.

"Gravity is gravity."

He was addressing me, but a dozen or so of my best friends had gathered around the game to follow our debate.

"Sure," I shrugged. "But sometimes we don't know what we don't know."

I nodded towards the taut net that divided the green slate between us.

"Let's say Pastor Ted is an ant. Ted is just a tiny little bug walking across this net. Let's say I decide to knock Ant Teddy off with a line-drive serve. From your point of view—as the ant—is the spinning ball that streaks towards you coming as a judgment from God? Or is it only a case of bad luck?"

I leaned forward. "The ant, certainly could never conceive that his meteor-of-doom was launched from a wooden paddle by a human being named Mark Hanson. The ant hasn't a clue. And he doesn't even realize he doesn't have a clue."

"If," said Ted, "it's your serve, then the ant hasn't got a worry in the world. To him, the ball is going to be a small white cloud high in the sky. An empty white dollop floating far overhead. Nothing to fear."

Everyone laughed.

"However, Mark, if you did somehow—against all odds—manage to hit Ant Teddy... then I suppose I would lose this round. I would finally have to believe in miracles."

More laughter.

"Ted, listen to what I'm saying. The ant doesn't know a ping pong ball from a cloud. We humans think we're smart, but we don't really know what's going on. Let alone why."

I shook my head. "For all we know, God and Satan are in the middle of a ping pong match. Maybe the latest tsunami in Indonesia is another line drive."

Angie smiled.

She told me once that I was brilliant. I'd been surprised when she'd used that word, but it had felt good. Fitting, even.

Angie was on the thin side, but her lively blonde hair and cautious laugh and perky charms kept me enthralled. I gave her a ride home from youth group every once in a while, and it always felt good to have her sitting next to me in my dad's car.

I beamed back at her beside the table, imaging my lips pressing into her smile. I nodded, resolving after the game to offer her another ride.

Ted tapped the edge of his paddle onto the table.

"Thousands of years ago," he said, "you'd be right. We were as clueless as ants. Today, though, we know all about tsunamis. Scientists know exactly what generates a tidal wave, and we can predict things like storms and tsunami landfalls with amazing accuracy."

He tapped the table twice more, lightly.

"We don't need to resort to explaining storms as battles between God and Satan. We don't need King Neptune to account for big waves. We know what makes lightning. We don't need a Zeus to throw magic spears from heaven."

"Maybe," I said, "even our best scientists don't know what they don't know."

"They know enough. In modern times, when properly understood, we realize miracles no longer happen... at least not in the ways people used to think."

He glanced at the others. "Dig deep enough, and there's always a logical explanation for everything."

Angie shifted. "What about love?" she asked. She glanced back and forth between Ted and me. "Last year, Mrs. Holmes told us that love is supernatural. She said love is a precious gift from God. A mystery nobody will ever really understand."

Ted hesitated.

"Even love," he finally sighed.

He took a deep breath. "It's a matter of biology. And behavioral conditioning, chemistry—pheromones.

The answers are there for anyone smart enough—and courageous enough—to dig all the way down to find them. The truth is there. And it's a treasure that's worth the dig."

"Truth?" I asked. "Yours, or mine? I choose to believe miracles are real."

"Miracles are wonderful surprises," he said, "but the laws of nature don't bend. Miracles cease to be magic—and can become even more breathtaking—once they are properly understood."

"Tell me," I demanded, squeezing the ball and raising my paddle. "When Moses held up his stick—and then parted the sea. How is that to be 'properly understood'?"

I aimed the paddle at Pastor Ted. "And what about Jesus with those sardines and bagels—feeding 5,000 fans out of practically nothing?"

My arm looped back, then snapped at the ball like an uncoiling snake. The spinning ball barely touched on Ted's side before shooting sideways far beyond his delayed and awkward swat.

Whoops of laughter erupted.

Angie retrieved the ball and walked it back to us, glancing between me and Ted, wondering whose turn it was to serve. I held out my hand. She stepped closer and pressed it into my palm, then melted back with a sheepish grin.

"Tell me again," I smiled. "Explain how those events didn't break the laws of nature."

Ted gently bumped the bridge of his little glasses. He glanced around the basement, taking inventory of who was within earshot. Finally, he dropped his paddle at the other end of the table.

"The wind blew," he said. "The wind explains the parting of the sea... just like it explains that lucky serve of yours."

He smirked through the giggles, then stepped to the wall and dipped a hand into the big red cooler. He fished around in the ice and retrieved a can of diet cola.

"Read your Bible, Mark. The Bible says Moses stood flapping in a bit of a hurricane. Exodus 14:21 spells it all out. If you were a Jew, the blasting gale was a miracle."

His can popped with a cracking *pfst*.

"But," he said, "from Pharaoh's side of the sea, it wasn't a miracle at all. What Pharaoh saw was a lucky reversal of weather for the Hebrews... and a dang unfortunate bit of tragedy for a legion of his finest charioteers."

He took a shallow sip.

"Hmm. Maybe." I could feel Angie leaning ever so slightly towards the conversation. Towards what I would say next.

"If the water was shallow right there in front of Moses, then maybe the right sort of wind might do it. I can see a way it could happen." I bounced the ball a couple times, then caught it midair.

"Okay," I asked, "and what about the fishes and loaves? How do you explain meat and bread popping into baskets from out of thin air?"

"Same thing."

Ted took a longer swig.

"Jesus was a great teacher. Probably the greatest motivational speaker of all time. When he held up the little boy's sack lunch and challenged his fans to share, they dug deep into their pockets and rummaged through their fanny packs. They obligingly pulled out whatever they could find."

He took another drink. "Crackers and cheese, old candy bars, gray wads of chewed gum rolled in dirty napkins."

We all laughed.

"Folks got so carried away and generous, pretty soon everyone had their fill. Especially of the gum—folks got their fill of those stale gum wads in a hurry."

"I'm not buying it," I said.

"Of course not. We haven't turned it into a miracle yet."

He put the soda down.

"For who-knows-how-many days after the picnic, everybody kept buzzing about how cool it all was. Over time, their stories grew. The bigger they told the story, the more important they sounded to everyone who hadn't been there to check the facts. Pretty soon, they all saw themselves as players in maybe the greatest flash mob picnic of all time." He grinned. "And there you have your miracle."

"Bullshit," I said.

Several of the younger kids winced, not sure whether that word was on the hit list or not.

"Your version doesn't add up." I said. "Jews didn't start chewing gum in Israel until after Constantine in the 4th century."

My crew erupted like I'd scored another ace. I studied Ted's eyes, assessing whether he appreciated my smart-mouthed tenacity, or if he was worried about losing control of the meeting.

He reached again for his drink.

"Ted," I pressed, "What you say makes sense. But do you really think hungry people would have called it a miracle if they knew it was only just food from their own knapsacks... and not a supernatural multiplication from the hand of God?"

"You tell me," he sighed, scratching his temple with the dry corner of his can. "You know the masses. You watch the news. Weak, simple-minded folks are desperate for sensations and mysteries. They love to stretch a story. They want to believe they've been blessed. Am I right... or what?"

"So, no miracles?"

Ted didn't quite have the chops to seal the deal. Or maybe he worried that if word got out he was a trasher of miracles, his debunking habits might cost him his job.

"Mark, it's not for me to say. You're holding court tonight as the brightest kid in the room. It's your call... genius."

I liked that.

The sound of it had a satisfying ring.

Genius.

36 CONSIDERING ANOTHER DAY

Freak slammed the door to his room upstairs.

Andy shook his head at me, then deserted the kitchen and strode to the game room, presumably to resume organizing maps, charts and notes he and Wilcox continuously shuffled and re-dealt atop the green billiard felt.

I joined Steve and Heather with my fourth beer on the couch.

"Freak," I sighed. "What an ego. He doesn't want a friend, he wants a minion."

We turned up the volume and watched more breaking news from the Petaluma earthquake. We tracked the latest updates about the storm developing off the California coast. Gradually, while the rest of the nation escalated, my heart slowed and my breathing returned to normal.

After a half hour the stories began repeating, and Steve killed the sound.

"What a mess," he said. "Do you think Freak is right? Is the Bay Area going to get slammed with more earthquakes... maybe even LA?"

"Who knows," I shrugged. "At least he hasn't predicted any disasters for Colorado yet. Has he?"

Steve laughed. "As far as I know, not yet."

Heather hugged what had become her favorite pillow. "Let's not wait. That man," she nodded towards the abandoned makeshift studio set over by the fireplace," he's mentally unstable. All of this talk about earthquakes and the end of the world...."

I gently removed her pillow.

"We have agreed," I said, "about staying through the weekend. Yes, he might be crazy. But who knows? After this morning's earthquake, all I am asking from you is for one more day. Not even the whole weekend. By this time tomorrow...."

"But," she whined, "I heard you two shouting in the kitchen. One minute you talk like he's your best friend. And then the next minute, you two are at each other's throats. There's no way you two will ever be able to work together for more than five minutes on anything."

Hmm.

She pressed the heel of her hand against her brow.

"I'm going to lay down for a few minutes. Would you mind bringing me some aspirins or something? I don't know what I did with my purse."

"I think it's in my room. Your room."

"Whatever," she mumbled. I helped her to her feet.

We found the missing purse. It was stuffed in her daisy daypack, and her pill case was inside the purse, almost empty. Within minutes the lights were out, and I left her with eyelids closed, a comforter tucked beneath her chin.

"She's nice," whispered Steve. "A little silly, but cute in her own way."

"No need to whisper," I said. "Heather can't hear you. Even if she could, she wouldn't remember later anyway. She passes out like this all the time."

"That's got to be a challenge," said Steve.

"Not really. Heather can be a lot of fun when she's been drinking. The trick is to catch her just before she goes over the edge. I know the signs."

"Anyway," said Steve. "I can see why you fell in love with her."

Hmm.

"So, Steve," I asked, changing the subject only a little, "have you ever been married... or anything like that?"

"No way. A few dates once in a while. Mostly from the Internet. Girls think it sounds cool that I work in television. But my relationships never really go anywhere."

I smiled encouragement. "There's nothing wrong with quick flips," I said. "We're both way too young to think about settling down."

Steve finished the last of his beer.

"I'd be happy to settle down." He placed his bottle on its side below the table, beside several others on the carpet near his foot.

"But," I said, "once you've got an old lady, you'd never be able to get away with a week like this. Heather has been giving me hell, and we're not even engaged."

"Well," chuckled Steve, "you've got to admit, she walked in on a pretty wild scene."

"Who do you think took it worse," I asked, "Heather... or Saundra?"

Steve stroked his chin for a moment. "Now that you mention it, I kinda know Saundra pretty well, and I think you're right. She was jealous, too."

"As well she should be," I laughed. "For once, I do believe Saundra has got some competition in the hottie department. Both Heather and Krissy."

"Oh, yeah," he grinned. "And guess who stopped by while you were out with Heather on your walk?"

"No way."

"That's right. But she was with her boyfriend. A big guy, by the way. Krissy came around to show him off... and to pick up her phone."

"Her phone?"

"Right. I guess someone must have moved it. Last night I put it on the counter, over by the napkin basket. But it wasn't there this morning. We finally found it on the table over against the wall."

Steve nodded at the decorative vase with a barren twig arrangement on the stand by the door to my room.

Heather's room.

Oops.

37
CENSORED
RAVINGS

I decided not to bother Heather, and I took my nap on the couch.

The next thing I knew, Wilcox was poking me awake and kicking Steve's foot. He handed Steve a napkin to wipe the drool from his couch-creased cheek, and then he instructed me to tuck in my shirt. In back, too.

"Pull yourselves together, boys," he said. "It's almost time for the Freak and Saundra show. And we're expecting guests."

He turned on the television, raised the volume, and scrolled to Channel 5.

"Mark," he asked, "do you want to wake Heather, or do you want to let her sleep it off?"

I tried to focus. I replayed the tape of what Wilcox had just said. I found myself torn between attending to the question of who our guests might be, versus what Wilcox was asking about Heather.

Hmm. I rubbed my neck. Another night on the couch was out of the question.

"We should let her sleep," I said at last. "Heather went down very tired, and she is pretty upset by all of this end-of-the-world talk."

"Right. Tired and upset. By the way, let me know if she runs out of aspirin. We've got a new freshly stocked first aid kit on the pool table in the war room. I had Andy pick one up... for all of these end-of-the-world emergencies you keep running into."

Wilcox handed me a white plastic garbage bag and pointed at the beer bottles strewn around the couch.

"And you'd better pick those up before Freak comes down. After falling from the clouds without a parachute, it'd be a shame if he broke his neck trying to step around a coffee table."

I took the bag and started hunting down the empties.

"So," I said, "you said something about guests."

"Saundra called," said Wilcox, heading to the kitchen. "She's really worried about how Freak is going to react to the final edit job her producer did on her interview. She figures she'd better be sitting with Freak when the bomb drops, so she can make her apologies and try to explain. She's afraid Freak's going to dump her and look for some other reporter to take her place. She knows plenty of competitors who are already licking their lips."

Hmm.

I found the last bottle. Not knowing there was one last swallow, I picked it up wrong and couldn't correct my grip before spilling a small splash onto the carpet. I flashed a guilty eye check in Steve's direction.

He winked, then reached over and tried to help by dabbing his napkin at the brown stain. Not much help.

From my knees, I noticed several more food and beverage ghosts of various shapes emerging from the carpet around the couch. I judged them all to be recent kills.

"Steve," I whispered, pointing at the darkest stain. "I remember the knife... but I can't remember what we did with the body."

Wilcox cleared his throat.

It was getting so I could feel the disapproval of Wilcox without even needing to look.

I did anyway. Wilcox had wandered back from the kitchen with a bowl of fruit, and he was now staring down from behind the couch.

"Funny you should ask," I said, regaining my feet. "For some reason, I'm craving white wine for tonight. Maybe we'll all be drinking non-staining whites and waters for the rest of our stay."

He shook his head.

I grinned. "How does that sound to you, Agent Wilcox... shall we save Uncle Sam some carpet cleaning fees by drinking the house white tonight... and water for you, of course?"

He passed me the bowl in exchange for my clanking bag of empties, then he returned to the kitchen without a word.

"By the way," I called, "I know Saundra and Freak both appreciate an occasional chilled Chardonnay, but what about our other guests... what will they be drinking tonight? You made it sound like we might be entertaining more than Saundra and Freak for the news."

Wilcox didn't answer. From the way he rattled a countertop pile of silverware and glasses into the sink, I deduced that at least one of our visitors might be his boss.

Ten minutes to five, the guests began to arrive.

Pastor Freak descended from his room, then Saundra in from the media truck, and then finally Sheriff Andy arrived in uniform... with a stout, balding government agent at his side. In seriously thick glasses.

The suited stranger was a bit of a disappointment—I had begun to hope against odds that Wilcox's unnamed guest might be Krissy. Heather was still asleep, and Saundra was sitting alone on a big chair to the side, looking very tense. It would have been nice to have Krissy to flirt with over the fresh beer I'd just pulled from the kitchen.

But Kristen didn't show up until after Saundra's interview was over; she arrived in a related story at the bottom of the hour.

The round guy didn't say much.

Not even his real name. We were all invited to simply call him Bud. Or Buddy. Or Mr. Buddy Bud. I got a little confused.

Mr. B wanted to shake Freak's hand and to watch the interview with us in silence. He mostly had come to huddle with Andy and Wilcox in the war room after the news ended. He feigned a passing interest in me, no interest in Steve, and a brief lingering interest in Saundra's skirt.

Saundra adjusted her legs.

Then came the Denver news.

Freak's interview got the big tease up front, but the hour's lead stories focused on a growing concern about aftershocks around the California earthquake, another alarmingly bad day on Wall Street, and another big Canadian snow storm bearing down on Colorado. Chain laws were expected to go into effect for numerous mountain passes within the next 24 hours.

"Wilcox," I said, pointing my beer at the weather map. "I hope you remembered to roll up the windows on my Hummer."

Steve was the only one to even grin.

I quietly put my bottle on the table and decided to slow down.

The Freak and Saundra show was delayed until after the first break. Their interview came up with a few arresting voiceover lines from Saundra while footage rolled of the two celebrities mouthing empty conversation from their fireside thrones. Steve's makeshift studio backdrop looked disarmingly cozy. Freak was positioned in his regal chair at a creative angle to accentuate the rounded boulders of the fireplace, complemented perfectly by Saundra's lovely profile.

I turned from the interview and glanced across the stone-faced live Saundra to the hearth and chimney masonry at the other end of our room. I needed to confirm that those really were the same smooth river rocks as seen on the screen.

Then we all settled or leaned forward as the voiceover faded and the censored give-and-take banter of the interview began.

In short, it was short.

For those of us expecting a big strawberry banana split with hot fudge, crushed nuts, whipped cream and a cherry on top... all we got was one half dollop of vanilla.

Freak excused himself.

He promised to return soon, which he did.

"What happened?" he asked, his voice flat.

Saundra cleared her throat.

"I did what I could," she said. "My producer was getting tremendous pressure from higher up."

"That's not the interview I gave," he said. "Not even close."

"I warned you," said Saundra. "I told you some of your quotes were never going to make the cut...."

"Some?"

They locked, unblinking, apparently prepared to work out some of their issues without boring the rest of us with their words. I remembered engaging in the unblinking game with the Reverend Jacobs once myself, the first time I tried to talk with him in the hospital. If I was a betting man, which I am, I'd put my money on something else. Not against either of these two pros.

Wilcox, perhaps feeling left out, broke the tie.

"Saundra. Freak. Knock it off."

They both turned at the same time.

He continued. "We're all on the same team here. Let's figure this out. Freak feels like he got cheated out of a chance to air his opinions. Saundra says she did the best she could."

"Not *opinions*," said Freak. "Prophecies. From the Lord. Critical information people needed to hear. Especially right now, tonight. My home is in the Bay Area. I've got friends there... seven million people have a *right* to know what's coming tomorrow. Good Friday is going to be hell."

He turned to Saundra.

"Do you think the networks will even bother to pick this up... or is Denver as far as this gutless-wonder is ever going to flop?"

Saundra winced. As pretty as she was, she still looked as if she'd been thrown under a bus... as if one wheel had bumped over, and the next big black tire was bearing down so fast she would never be able to roll clear from its path.

Andy stood.

"Freak is right," he said, addressing Saundra, and then Wilcox. "If there is even a remote chance Freak might be correct about what is coming, then people need to be prepared. If not the general public, then at least the regional emergency support teams and all of the local first responders."

Andy turned to the stranger. "Bud, how prepared are they right now?"

Mr. B tapped the bridge of his glasses.

"Everyone is already on high alert. There is nothing more they can do. The Petaluma quake triggered protocols in California and set things in motion on every level... we are all prepared for every contingency."

He turned to Freak. "Thank you, Reverend Jacobs, for your civic-minded concern. Your views have been relayed to all interested parties, from the teams on the ground around the Bay all the way up to President, who has shown considerable interest in you."

Hmm.

Andy sat back down.

"The President," said Freak, "does not share my point of view on almost anything. He has made that clear in the past. My message does not speak to FEMA politics, nor to disaster recovery models. In the coming days, we will be rapidly moving beyond the capacity of crisis response teams and federal emergency assistance. My message is for the people, and it speaks to matters far beyond just fixing porch swings and issuing tax rebates for millionaires who want to refit their damaged roofs with solar panels."

He slowed, shuddered. "You have no idea what I've seen."

"We all," said Wilcox, "have imagined such nightmares. Let us hope...."

"Not dreams," Freak said. "Visions of what is to be. Even the task of burying the dead... many tens of thousands.... America has never seen anything close to the likes of this before. Most of us haven't got a clue...."

Eventually, Saundra broke the silence.

"I'm sorry, Freak," she said. "Maybe if something actually happens in San Francisco tomorrow, then perhaps the station will allow us to do another interview...."

"No!" said Freak.

This time everyone winced.

"I'm not," continued Freak, "going to waste another day with Channel 5. I think it's time for a free-market press conference. I'll let the competition for ratings determine who gives this message the exposure it demands...."

"Slow down, champ," said Wilcox. "You can't just...."

"What I really need," said Freak, "is to regain some control over the message. I need to get back on top of this before it's too late."

"What are you thinking?" I asked.

"I want my own show again. I need to get back on the air, uncensored. Tomorrow, or as soon as possible. I need to buy an hour of uninterrupted airtime. By Easter Sunday... at the latest."

I had forgotten we were sliding into Easter weekend.

"Saundra," he said, suddenly hopeful. "Can you help me with that? Might it be possible for us to film an edition of *The Final Hour* here in Colorado? You're still my first choice for this. But unless you can help me here, you and I may have to go our own ways."

"Please," she said, "I do want to help you. I've actually come to like you. And I do believe what you have to share is important. It's not fair, though, if you're going to coerce or blackmail me into meeting demands...."

"Ms. Paige," he snapped. "By now, there are other stations and other networks who will be more than willing to work with me. I've already heard commentators from the right—and from the left—complaining about the monopoly Channel 5 is perceived to be holding over me and over this story. Reporters have hinted at possible improprieties. Issues of the free press. Your days of controlling all of the exclusive interviews has come to an end...."

"Freak," said Wilcox. "Don't be so sure about what you can pull off. If you walk out of here, or if you start talking to other venues, you might discover yourself being considerably more censored and marginalized than you already are."

"Is that a threat, Agent Wilcox?"

"No threat. I'm just reminding you, as you've already heard, that people are following you and your interviews closely... all the way up the ladder to Washington. I have been in contact with several executives with Saundra's network, and—at least for now—you will continue to have access to the airwaves. But if you try to go rogue, then I can make no promises as to what your broadcasting future may hold."

Freak paused. He closed his eyes and tried to collect himself. He touched two fingers to the top of his scar, held them there for a moment, and then traced a ridge down to his chin.

"Wilcox, I hear you. I can appreciate your job and the position you are in. But I cannot—nor can the world—afford to play any more political games with this information. Millions of lives are at stake."

His gaze swept the room. "The sand is getting low in the hourglass, and yet nobody seems to care."

"People care," said Wilcox. "And we care about you and your opinions. But national hysteria—let alone global anarchy—are in nobody's interest. My men are running down some leads on the group that might be behind what happened at the tree. They call themselves The Sons of Thor. They're a new outlaw group of White Supremacists, and they've been building an arsenal, moving around, trying to stay off the grid. We know very little about them except they are very dangerous. And for some whacked-out reason, if their web site and blogs are any indication, they see you as an insult or threat to their cause."

"If they *are* evil," said Freak, "then I *should* be a threat to them. But as long as I remain without a voice, and as long as I am locked up in this suite, I am not a threat to anyone. Nobody needs to fear me... no matter how dangerous or bad they may be."

"As you know," said Wilcox. "I'm on your side. I have dedicated my life to fighting evil people. I want to help you, to be a sounding board and a resource for you. And I want to make sure you are safe. You've got some folks here around you right now who are professionals. You've got a seasoned team of experts at your disposal, folks who are willing to work with you to keep things from getting out of hand...."

"Out of hand?" Freak glared. "Are you kidding? Have you not heard a thing I've said since you arrived?"

"Your television show," I asked, "do you still have a spot this weekend reserved... or whatever it is you would need in order to be able to broadcast? I have no idea how these things work, but I think...."

"Mark," said Wilcox. "Don't go there. It's not going to happen."

"Hold on," I said. "The last time I checked, this was still America. We still have a Constitution that clearly...."

Saundra stood and crossed to Freak. Sat beside him.

"I'll do what I can," she said. "I've been trying to toe the line with everyone. But based upon what I'm picking up from Wilcox, I can see where this is going. And I don't like it."

She put a hand on his knee.

"But," she said, "if God really has chosen you, and if even a few of your prophecies are going to come true, then this is all in God's hands, right?"

Everyone waited.

"I'm with you, Freak," she said. "I've already put my career on the line by fighting with my boss on your behalf every day I've been on this story. You've had me thinking I've seen angels... and worse. You've had me praying in a chapel and pouring over my Bible for answers... or even for the right questions to ask. And now, you've convinced me. Either this whole thing is a random farce, or... God is in control."

She squeezed his knee.

"Come on, Freak," she implored. "Is God in this, or not?"

Freak studied Saundra's eyes.

I studied Saundra's hand.

As time stood still, I became increasingly aware of where her hand was extended across her hemline, where her skirt had slipped up above her knee when she sat down. I began to wonder how long she was going to leave those slender fingers wrapped on his leg, where their knees touched. Tiny electric gnats began buzzing within my skull....

"Yes," he said at last.

Finally, she removed her hand and I could breathe again.

"Saundra," he said, smiling for the first time all evening. "You are right. This belongs to God."

Freak turned to me, apparently with no idea about what I'd just been forced to endure.

"Mark, we need to trust God on this. He has a plan."

"Right," I sighed. "If you say so."

"Saundra," said Freak. "In our first interview, you asked me a question. It's something I've been thinking about and praying over ever since. You asked me what kind of prophet of doom I was."

"The question," she said, "was whether you were a Noah or a Jonah."

"Well," he said, "in all fairness, before you put any more on the line, you need to know my answer."

"And?"

"I still don't know." Freak lifted his head and swept the room. "All I know is what I've seen for the coming months, and it is bad. Really bad for millions...."

He turned back to Saundra. "But God has not yet shown me how it ends. And until it ends, I won't know if I'm a Noah or a Jonah. Whether a flood of total destruction entirely clears the slate, or whether the world turns before it burns. Lord, have mercy."

"Thanks," she said. "You're not making me feel any better, but I needed to know. I really am sorry about tonight's interview. I wish there was something else I could still do...."

"You tried." Freak patted her knee.

I tried to look away, but couldn't. Thankfully, he dropped his hand almost immediately and stood.

"And Saundra, you reminded me about who is in control." Freak lowered his gaze to me.

"Mark, if God could drop me safely into your backyard and bring us to where we are right now, he certainly will not let the Devil stop the word of the Lord from going forth according to his sovereign will tonight... in time to warn those who need to know. But it looks like we're in for a long night of prayer."

"Right," I sighed.

"Impossible," said Andy. "Channel 5 has the footage, and they've already made the call to censor your predictions. You can pray all you want, but your warnings will never get out tonight. This round of the story is dead."

Freak lifted a hand from where he stood, then closed his eyes.

"Lord," he called, "have mercy. We trust you, Jesus. We serve you. And we cry out for the people of California. Have your way, Lord. Let no schemes of Satan thwart your sovereign plans. May your grace and truth be known. We...."

"Holy Cow!" shouted Steve, pointing at the screen. "Turn it up!"

38
WORD ON THE STREET

"... and once again, standing live beside me, I have Pastor Rodney Gilford, religious leader of the Blue River Bible Church."

Channel 5's reporter Tom Jackson appeared to be gloating. According to Saundra, Tom always appeared to be gloating.

But Gilford looked different.

Less full of himself. Nervous, but happy.

"Pastor Gilford," urged Tom, "tell us more about what happened here yesterday at your church."

Gilford glanced at the camera, then back to Tom.

"Well, as I said before, Reverend Jacobs came here to pray. He came into my church."

Gilford threw a thumb low over his shoulder, across the milling crowd and the packed parking lot toward the familiar white steeple.

"I have to admit," he continued, "at first, I didn't know what to think about the man. I've never been around celebrities prior to yesterday, and now all of a sudden...."

"Tell us," said Tom, "about the miracle."

"Well, as I said before, while we were trying to pray, all of a sudden Reverend Jacobs zeroed in on me. It was like he could see right into me. He said he knew I had cancer. He even knew what kind and how much...."

"What type of cancer did you have, Pastor Gilford?"

"Well... it's kinda embarrassing." He shifted legs. "I had colon cancer. Bad. It was killing me. The doctors were trying to be optimistic, but I could tell deep down, because of the way it was spreading and everything, they pretty much had given up on any sort of a recovery...."

"And then what happened?"

"I had been praying all along, of course, ever since the prognosis turned south. My wife was praying. The whole church was praying. We'd all been praying for months...."

"Until yesterday," asked Tom. "Is that right?"

"That is correct. Reverend Jacobs stood up in the church and walked toward me. He said the Lord had heard all of those prayers, and God wanted to heal me. Right then and there. And then he did. Through Reverend Jacobs, the Lord seems to have healed me. Amen!"

Several people nearby murmured enthusiastic approvals.

"And how do you know this? Have you been able to confirm...."

"Oh, yes." Gilford beamed. "As it turns out, I already had a doctor's appointment on my calendar for this morning. It's been confirmed and double checked. They did all kinds of tests. As far as the doctors can tell, the cancer is all gone...."

A handful of Gilford's family and friends shouted muffled hurrahs and praises.

"My wife was so excited," said Gilford, "she started calling church people before we even got home. The whole church knew within an hour."

"Yesterday," said Tom, "you and I stood in this same parking lot. At that time, you had some pretty harsh words for Bill Jacobs. You insinuated that perhaps he could not be trusted. And then you also leaked to the media some footage showing his scars."

"Well," said Gilford, looking down, and then up directly into the camera. "Today, I'd just like to say how sorry I am. I was scared, and I believed I was dying. And I felt so much power flowing in that man, I jumped to the conclusion maybe he was evil or something. I'm not sure I've ever been around anyone with power like that before."

"You accused him of having the Mark of the Beast."

"Well, not exactly, but something like that."

Gilford licked his lips.

"If you're watching this, Reverend Jacobs, I just want you to know how sorry I am...."

I tore my eyes from the television and glanced at Freak.

He was trembling.

"San Francisco," pressed Tom. "Tell us about San Francisco."

"Okay," Gilford turned back to the reporter. "Yesterday, when he was praying for San Francisco, I couldn't really understand what the Reverend was saying. Like I said, I was afraid maybe he was wicked or something. But then, right there in the waiting room at the doctor's office today, the television news started showing stuff about the earthquake. And then I knew."

"Knew what?"

"That Reverend Jacobs must be a prophet. That God seems to have called him to speak to the world. That the Lord has a message for us, and this man needs to be heard."

People cheered from on and off the shot. The bearded Elder David Bates leaned into the frame, clapping, thumbs up.

"Yesterday," said the reporter, "you said people needed to choose."

Gilford smiled. "Yes. I said that. And I stick by it."

"So then, what does that mean to you today?"

"I still think people do need to choose. People need to choose to listen to this man of God and to hear him out. We need to test his words. He could be wrong about some of it. But we do need to listen."

"Pastor Gilford, what do you say to the critics who believe Reverend Jacobs is just a very smart man? That he studies history and science and psychology—that he does his homework—and then he simply makes statistically probable guesses."

"Huh?"

"Well, for example, he lives in the Bay Area. For many years, he probably has been reading everything he can about earthquakes and how they act and what is likely to happen. So when he says something about earthquakes, he is more likely repeating the opinions and predictions of experts rather than hearing something from God."

"I wouldn't know about that," said Gilford. "All I can tell you is... I was as good as dead, and now I'm feeling very much alive."

"In your opinion, then: prophet or fraud?"

"Are you kidding?" laughed Gilford. "God is using that man!"

"We have someone else of interest here," said Tom, "but before we talk to her, I'd like you to tell us about all of these cars here tonight in your church parking lot."

Gilford grinned.

He wheeled around away from the camera and snapped his thumb up in a victory salute, hoisting it as high in the air as he could reach, waving it towards the steeple.

Immediately, a small roar of clapping and cheers arose from those milling about the front of the chapel.

And the bell began to ring. Loudly.

"We're here," Gilford shouted into the camera over the din, "to celebrate. To give thanks to the Lord for healing me... for the miracle...." Gilford choked slightly, and then awkwardly stepped back. Within moments he had disappeared into the crowd.

"Also with us live," said Tom, "we have Miss Kristen LaBette."

The camera pulled wider and Krissy stepped into the frame. She quickly made her way tight to Tom Jackson, leaning close, stretching her bubbling smile into the microphone.

"Hi," she said. "It's so cool to be doing this."

"Miss LaBette," said Tom, "we're live on Channel 5 News."

"I know," Krissy giggled, loud enough to be heard over the tolling bell. "This is so cool."

"When our Channel 5 team arrived here an hour ago," said Tom, "while we were setting up our live remote truck, Kristen, you left from your job as a clerk at the Last Stop Liquor Store and walked over here to talk with me."

"Yes," she said. "I figured you were doing another story, and I thought you'd want to know some more stuff about Freak."

I noticed she was wearing a bright new T-shirt. It looked familiar.

"You refer to Reverend Jacobs as... 'Freak'?"

"Right. Everyone who knows him does. I've met him, you know. I've been to the place where he is staying. That's what he likes to have people to call him. *Freak*."

"Yes. And what is it you have learned about him?"

"First, I want to say thank you to my friend, Mark Hanson." She waved at the camera. "Hi, Mark!"

She turned back to Tom and said something I missed.

I glanced around the room and caught Steve's grin. Freak didn't turn, but he shook his head—up and down for a change, instead of his usual back and forth.

"It was Mark who gave me some really cool footage of Freak. He put it on my cell phone." She pried her phone free from her back pocket and showed it to the camera.

This time everyone—including both Agent Wilcox and Mr. B—turned to look at me. I shrugged an "I have no idea what she's talking about," then motioned everyone back to the story.

"Kristen," said Tom, "you did not mention you had a video when we talked a few minutes ago before going on the air. I was under the impression you had gathered all of your information from a conversation that you had overheard...."

"Oh, no, it's all on film. It's already on my new website. I made this new website called FreakFall.com. My boyfriend and I plan to put all kinds of cool stuff up on the website really soon. Stuff to watch, and stuff to buy."

"Like this shirt that you're wearing?"

"Right. This one is a prototype we whipped up using acrylics. But we're going to be silk screening and printing more of these in all different sizes all weekend. People can order these and lots of other stuff at our website, FreakFall.com."

I took a quick peek at Saundra. I knew it was a live feed, but I assumed it was airing with a few seconds of delay. I was a little surprised they were letting Krissy promote her for-profit website so freely.

Saundra's face gave away nothing but profound fascination... with both Tom Jackson, and with the equally ever-astonishing Miss Krissy.

"Kristen," said Jackson, lowering his gaze. "I like your shirt. But I'm still trying to figure it out. Could you please explain it for our viewers."

"Sure," she said, pulling the bottom away from her waist so she could look down and see it.

"We wrote 'Freak Power' on it because we think Freak is amazing. The stuff he says will blow your mind. And because he couldn't be killed, even in an exploding airplane and everything, we figure he really has some sort of mystical energy or something."

"So, having met him, do you think he actually has supernatural powers?"

"Sure. I guess. I don't know how his powers work, though. It's crazy, but when we started designing my shirt this afternoon, we hadn't even heard yet about the power he has to do miracles... like healing cancer from the pastor over at the church yesterday."

"And," said Tom, "please explain the picture."

"Of course. The round yellow head is the famous 'smile' face everybody already knows. But you'll see here," she pointed to the red patch on one cheek, "this is Freak's scar."

"Very clever."

"Do ya think? We got the idea this morning when I went to get my phone from Mark at the lodge in Breckenridge. That's where Freak and Mark and everyone is staying. There was a man outside of the lodge, and he was holding a sign. His sign had a face on it kinda like this one, and that's where we got the idea."

"And why is his smile all curvy... waving up and down like that?"

"Because Freak is smiling, and he is sad at the same time. That is the way Freak is if you get to know him. He is always happy, and always sad at the same time. When you see my website and watch the video clips, you'll understand more about why he is always like that."

"Kristen, I have not seen your video, so perhaps you can summarize for us?"

"Okay, sure. Freak says one side of his face is healthy, and that side represents 'mercy.' Or maybe it was 'grace.' I forget which Bible word he used. Anyway, one side symbolizes all of the happy love God has for everybody in the world."

"What about the scar?"

"That's the hard part. Freak says God gave him the scars to tell the world everything is not always all happy. Sometimes there is evil and pain. His scars are a symbol for the harshness of the truth. Freak says God is love... and at the same time, God is also truth. Happy, and sometimes sad, all in one. Mind blowing, huh?"

She glanced again briefly at her shirt, then back to Tom.

"Freak says all of the horrible disasters he is predicting are going to be very ugly, like his scars. But he says the terrible stuff is what sometimes comes when you get the truth."

Tom darted a quick look past the camera, apparently toward the remote truck or someone off screen. He touched his earphone for a moment.

"Just one more minute, Kristen. You said Mark Hanson gave you some video footage of Freak talking?"

"That's right. The film was pretty long, and some of it was shaky and pointing down and everything, so we broke it all up into some pretty good short clips. Did I mention we also posted all of the video clips on Facebook and YouTube?"

"No," said Tom. "But tell us more."

"Mark recorded it all during when Saundra Paige was talking to Freak at the lodge for her Channel 5 interview...."

Hmm.

Heather! Heather must have been recording on Krissy's phone....

"During the interview, Freak said a lot of things. He made a lot of prophecies... you know, predictions about how San Francisco was going to be completely destroyed tomorrow, and horrible things like that. He also said that besides the total collapse of San Francisco, the earthquake would spread down and destroy Los Angeles, and Seattle was going to get flattened by a tsunami...."

"Excuse me, Kristen. Did you say Freak predicted...."

Technical difficulties disrupted the live feed.

A commercial break immediately filled the dead air.

But it was too late.

Clips from the FreakFall.com website and YouTube were already downloading, being reposted and going viral before anyone could get a fat finger in the dike.

The word was on the street.

Epilogue

When I finally fell asleep, Freak was still praying.

Spellbound, most of us had watched the news for hours. Heather came out of her room at one point for some food. She found out what was going on, watched for a few minutes over my shoulder, started shaking, then disappeared. The rest of us continued to surf the networks deep into the night as more and more of Freak's censored remarks found their way from social media sites into mainstream television newscasts and special programming.

Earlier in the day, several cable stations had committed to continuous coverage of the Petaluma earthquake disaster. Freak's fireside apocalyptic predictions for the Bay Area reenergized their broadcasts at the very moment in the evening when they were running low on fresh material. Additionally, the new Freak clips provided a legitimate excuse for them to resurrect dramatic highlights from their previous in-depth coverage of the Falling Skies attacks.

By prime time, even Channel 5 had begun airing and dissecting "over the top" quotes and "off the record" snippets of the viral clips from Saundra's interview.

The buzz and the editorializing over the catastrophic prophecies Heather had recorded on Krissy's camera phone quickly escalated into a global roar.

And, according to Krissy, the underground footage could all be traced back to the bold and brilliant work of Mark Hanson, bulldog champion of the free press.

"It figures," Saundra sighed.

Eventually, the flat screen was black and the room was empty and quiet except for me, Freak, and a snoring Steve.

"Pandora's box," I whispered, pointing at the TV.

I reached for the switch and dimmed the lamp at my end of the couch.

"Not a pagan box," replied Freak, but heaven's warnings. From here to the end, the Seven Bowls will play big on the home screen."

"Tomorrow," I said, "you'll have to live with the consequences of what you unleashed today."

"I unleashed nothing," he sighed. "This is God's work. And not just me. The entire world will have to deal with what happens next."

Freak stood and glanced at the fireplace, where only hours ago he had predicted the fall of San Francisco and the beginning of the end.

"One more day," he asked, "right? You said you would give me one more day?"

"Yes. By this time tomorrow, I'll be totally in, or all out. Depending upon what happens in California, we'll both know where we stand."

"I already know where I stand," he sadly smiled. "You're the one who has got to make peace with his place in all of this... and with what is yet to come."

"Peace starts," I said, "with a good night of sleep." I kicked off my shoes and swung my feet around onto the couch.

He took two steps, then turned back.

"Would you mind," he asked, "if I go pray for a while... over by the fireplace? I felt God with me there this afternoon. Now God and I need to talk some more."

"Sure. Just keep it down as much as you can. I've decided to leave Heather alone again tonight. I'll be sleeping another night out here."

"I can see that." Freak reached over and picked up a couch pillow.

"Here," he said, gently tossing it my way. "Good call. Let her sleep."

His prayers were soft. Sometimes clear, sometimes indecipherable. Saundra might have been able to understand, but not me.

He seemed to be pleading. He sounded not at all eager for what he expected tomorrow to bring.

Myself, I'm not one to pray.

For the most part, I'm not a person who worries much about trying to change the course of history, or even my own plans for the next day. But as I closed my eyes and listened to the Reverend W.B. Jacobs sobbing, kneeling at the hearth, I began to seriously consider the possibility America might be headed for some serious shaking.

Perhaps even a bigger shaking beyond what Freak could see.

And then suddenly I knew. I don't know how, but I did. A wave of something sweet—and yet bitter—washed over me. It wasn't intuition or premonition. It was knowledge.

Freak was right about Good Friday. Easter weekend this year was going to be an awful time for the West Coast. But there was more.

Something bad was going to happen here in Colorado... at the lodge.

I felt a strange urge to go to Heather in the other room. To gently crawl into bed beside her. Not even to wake her. Just to hold her.

And then I pictured the keys to my beastie. I was going to need my keys.

Compared to what Freak was praying, it probably wasn't much. But as I fell asleep, I whispered my first prayer in many years:

Lord have mercy.

———— END BOOK I ————

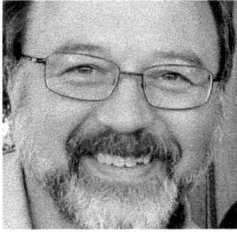

DAVE CHEADLE has published over 150 articles and five books, including the award-winning first volume of the Freak Trilogy, *Freak Fall*.

His fiction, social history research, and religious writing has appeared in St. Anthony Messenger, Cornerstone, The Church Herald, Sports Collectors Digest, and dozens of other venues. His first novel, *Family Ashes*, debuted 15 years ago as a Rocky Mountain Fiction Writers Colorado Gold finalist.

Cheadle's non-fiction works have appeared in publications ranging from Persimmon Hill to Victorian Decorating and Lifestyle Magazine. He has served as the managing editor for two nationally circulated collectibles magazines, and he is the author of the definitive work on 19th Century lithographed business advertising cards, *Victorian Trade Cards: Historical Reference and Value Guide*.

Cheadle has taught high school writing, photography, literature and history. In the 1980's his high school journalism program was recognized with the highest honors in the state of Colorado. In 1989 he led a team of high school newspaper editors to Germany–loaded with cameras and equipment from three Denver television stations–to provide live reporting on the collapse of the Berlin Wall.

He lives in Colorado where he founded and now leads the CenterPoint Missional Community movement in Denver. He is the father of two college graduates, and he has been married for 33 years.

For more information about *Freak Fall*, *Freak Unleashed*, or *Freak Ending*, or to order books, visit: www.FreakTrilogy.com.

www.ingramcontent.com/pod-product-compliance
Lightning Source LLC
Chambersburg PA
CBHW072045020426
42334CB00017B/1392